EATING HEALTHY EATING *Right*

SCOTT WILSON, C.E.C., A.A.C.
JODY WILKINSON, M.D.

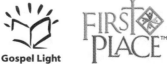

Gospel Light

FIRST PLACE™

Gospel Light is an evangelical Christian publisher dedicated to serving the local church. We believe God's vision for Gospel Light is to provide church leaders with biblical, user-friendly materials that will help them evangelize, disciple and minister to children, youth and families.

It is our prayer that this Gospel Light resource will help you discover biblical truth for your own life and help you minister to others. May God richly bless you.

For a free catalog of resources from Gospel Light, please contact your Christian supplier or contact us at 1-800-4-GOSPEL or www.gospellight.com.

PUBLISHING STAFF
William T. Greig, Chairman
Kyle Duncan, Publisher
Dr. Elmer L. Towns, Senior Consulting Publisher
Pam Weston, Senior Editor
Patti Pennington Virtue, Associate Editor
Jeff Kempton, Editorial Assistant
Hilary Young, Editorial Assistant
Bayard Taylor, M.Div., Senior Editor, Biblical and Theological Issues
Samantha A. Hsu, Cover and Internal Designer

ISBN 0-8307-3022-2
© 2002 First Place
All rights reserved.
Printed in the U.S.A.

Any omission of credits is unintentional. The publisher requests documentation for future printings.

CAUTION
The information contained in this book is intended to be solely informational and educational. It is assumed that the First Place participant will consult a medical or health professional before beginning this or any other weight-loss or physical-fitness program.

PRAISE FOR *EATING HEALTHY, EATING RIGHT*

Eating Healthy, Eating Right approaches healthy eating sensibly, and it provides a variety of foods that can easily be exchanged. This book provides great tools for professionals and those who are taking control of their health by choosing sensible foods and realistic portions. Meals will be refreshing with exciting colors, textures and flavors!

—Suzanne Magni, R.D., L.D.
Cooking School Manager
Healthy Cooking Instructor
Nutrition Educator

Eating Healthy, Eating Right is a keeper—not only for today's busy on-the-go workers but also nutritionists who need menu selections for their clients. It's like having your own personal chef advising you on healthful meal planning. Part of Chef Scott's culinary mastery is the ability to take the ordinary and, with a few simple additions, create an extraordinary, heart-healthy meal!

—Beverley Demetrius, M.A., R.D., L.D.
Nutrition Services Director
Cobb County Health Department
Marietta, Georgia

This book is an indispensable, delicious road map for planning the lifelong journey of eating healthy and eating right!

—Molly Gee, M.Ed., R.D., L.D.

Contents

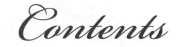

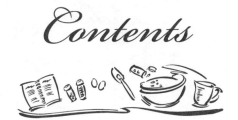

Contributors 9
Foreword by Marita Littauer 10
Introduction 11

Meal Planning Tools

Weekly Meal Planner 14
Sample Weekly Meal Planner 16
Eating Healthy, Eating Right Grocery List 18
Conversion Chart for Equivalent Imperial and Metric Measurements 20

Breakfasts

BREAKFAST MENUS

Cold Cereals 24
Hot Cereals 27
Continental Style 28
Grab 'n' Go 32
Pancakes and Waffles 33

BREAKFAST MENUS WITH RECIPES

French Toast, Pancakes and Waffles 35
Miscellaneous 37
Smoothies 39

Lunches

LUNCH MENUS

Dine In/Take Out 42

Frozen Entrées 44

Miscellaneous 46

Poultry and Seafood 48

Sandwiches 50

Soups and Salads 55

Quick Lunches 59

LUNCH MENUS WITH RECIPES

Cold Sandwiches 61

Hot Off the Grill 62

Miscellaneous 64

Salads 67

Dinners

DINNER MENUS

Dine In/Take Out 72

Frozen Entrées 74

DINNER MENUS WITH RECIPES

Beef 75

Pork 85

Poultry 88

Seafood 109

Vegetables and Pasta 120

Side Dishes

Potatoes 126
Salad Dressings 128
Salads and Slaws 129
Salsas 134
This 'n' That 135
Veggies 138

Healthy Living

BE PREPARED

Supermarket Guide: Solutions for Healthy Shopping 146
Stocking the Healthy Kitchen 148
Tools for a Healthy Kitchen 151

BE INFORMED

Understanding the Nutrition Facts Panel 154
Understanding Portion Control 157
Sweetness by Any Other Name 159
Convenience Foods—Making the Most of Your Time 162
Changing Recipes 164
Adding Flavor the Healthy Way 166
Meatless Meals 168
Off to a Good Start 171
Take Time for a Healthy Lunch 173
Outsmarting the Snack Attack 176
Healthy Snack Choices 178

EATING HEALTHY ON THE GO

Nutrition While Traveling 179
Life in the Fast-Food Lane 182
Dining Out Asian Style 184
Dining Out *Delizioso!* 186
Dining Out—South of the Border 189

AN OUNCE OF PREVENTION

The Truth About Fats 191
Choosing High-Fiber Foods 196
Understanding Vitamins and Minerals 199
Dietary Supplements—Miracle or Myth? 207
Preventing Cancer 210
Controlling Cholesterol 213
Preventing Diabetes 216

RECIPE INDEX

RECIPE INDEX 220

Contributors

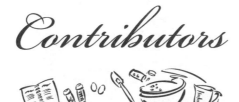

Scott Wilson, C.E.C., A.A.C., the author of the menu plans, has been cooking professionally for 23 years. A certified executive chef with the American Culinary Federation, he currently works in the Greater Atlanta area as a personal chef and food consultant and is a Certified Personal Chef with the United States Personal Chef Association. Along with serving as the national food consultant for First Place, he is on the culinary program advisory board of the Art Institute in Atlanta. Scott has also authored two cookbooks, *Dining Under the Magnolia* and *Healthy Home Cooking*. He is also active in church work and enjoys spending time with his wife of 18 years, Jennifer, and their daughter, Katie.

William J. (Jody) Wilkinson, M.D., M.S., the writer of many of the information sheets, is a physician and exercise physiologist at the Cooper Institute in Dallas, Texas. He did his medical training at the University of Texas Health Science Center in San Antonio, Texas and Baylor University Medical Center in Dallas. Dr. Wilkinson is the Director of The Cooper Institute Weight Management Research Center. He strongly believes in using biblical teaching to motivate people to take care of their physical bodies and enjoy abundant living. Jody and his wife, Natalie, have been married 10 years and have two daughters, Jordan and Sarah, and twin sons, Joel and Cooper.

Foreword

I am what is known as a "foodie." I *love* food—I love to plan it, cook it, serve it and eat it. Yet I believe in taking care of my body—the temple of God—and my health. I work at staying in shape through a combination of proper exercise and eating well.

I am also a proponent of a balanced life, knowing that we are made up of many parts. We need spiritual as well as physical nourishment. We need fellowship almost as much as we need food. It is for these reasons that I have appreciated my involvement with First Place over the past 15 years. This program incorporates these vital elements—and it works. While living a life of balance is easy for me, I know most of my friends share my love for eating but not for the planning and preparation that wise dining requires. For most of us, just getting the food on the table is enough without having to think through exchanges and calories, complications that can make eating healthy seem like an insurmountable task.

This is why *Eating Healthy, Eating Right* is such a valuable tool for the person who wants to lose weight (or keep in shape) while staying healthy. Reproducible menu-planning guides and grocery lists are included. Appropriate menus and recipes are featured for every meal from breakfast to dinner, every taste from simple to spicy and every lifestyle from fast-food to gourmet. Tips for stocking and organizing your kitchen will allow you to make healthy eating as easy as possible. Guides for dining out in virtually every type of restaurant allow you to share meals with friends and family and still eat right. To round out and complete the program, *Eating Healthy, Eating Right* even offers helpful advice on nutritional supplements and explores the connection between food and disease.

More than a cookbook, more than a diet book, *Eating Healthy, Eating Right* is the tool you need for eating healthy and eating right!

—Marita Littauer
President
CLASServices, Inc.
(Christian Leaders, Authors and Speakers Services)

Introduction

The recipes and menu plans in *Eating Healthy, Eating Right* were designed not only to complement the First Place weight-loss program but also for use by anyone interested in making healthier food and lifestyle choices.

All recipe and menu exchanges were determined using the MasterCook software, a program that accesses a database containing over 6,000 food items prepared using the United States Department of Agriculture (USDA) publications and information from food manufacturers. As with any nutritional program, MasterCook calculates the nutritional values of the recipes based on ingredients. Nutrition may vary due to how the food is prepared and where the food comes from (i.e., soil content, season, ripeness, processing and method of preparation). For these reasons, please use the recipes and menu plans as approximate guides. As always, consult your physician and/or a registered dietitian before starting a weight-loss program.

HOW THE EXCHANGES WORK

The menu plans in this book are based on approximately 1,400 calories per day. You will need to consult with a physician and/or a registered dietitian to determine your optimum daily calorie needs. For further information on food exchanges, contact the American Dietetic Association or the American Diabetes Association.

Breakfast	2 breads, 1 fruit, 1 milk[1], 0-½ fat
Lunch	2 meats, 2 breads, 1 vegetable, 1 fruit, 1 fat
Dinner	3 meats, 2 breads, 2 vegetables, 1 fat
Snacks	1 bread, 1 fruit, 1 milk, ½-1 fat (or any remaining exchanges)

If you are following a higher-calorie plan, add the following to your daily exchanges:

1,600 calories 2 breads, 1 fat
1,800 calories 2 meats, 3 breads, 1 vegetable, 1 fat
2,000 calories 2 meats, 4 breads, 1 vegetable, 3 fats
2,200 calories 2 meats, 5 breads, 1 vegetable, 1 fruit, 5 fats
2,400 calories 2 meats, 6 breads, 2 vegetables, 1 fruit, 6 fats

Note

1. When a meat exchange is used in a breakfast, the milk exchange is omitted.

HOW TO USE *EATING HEALTHY, EATING RIGHT*

This book has been arranged to help you make healthy, tasty choices as you plan your meals. Planning meals for the week will be a snap as you use the information provided.

MEAL PLANNING TOOLS

The Weekly Meal Planner

The handy, reproducible meal-planning chart on pages 14 and 15 has been designed to help you plan healthy balanced meals for the week and also to help you keep track of your exchanges. Whether you're following this program or the recipes in this book for weight loss or simply because of a desire to eat healthier, this chart can be a big help in reaching your goal. A completed sample has also been provided (pp. 16-17) to help you get started on a week's worth of menu planning!

The Grocery List

Once you've planned your menus for the week, you can use the reproducible grocery list on pages 18 and 19 to prepare for any shopping to be done to ensure you have what you need to make your meals. This will help not only in shopping for the items you'll need, but also to curb impulse purchases.

Conversion Chart for Equivalent Imperial and Metric Measurements
This conversion chart is provided to aid those who reside outside the United States in using this helpful resource for planning healthy meals.

THE MENUS AND RECIPES

The menus in each section—breakfast, lunch or dinner—provide a wide variety of meals that can be prepared at home. Also included are ideas for using frozen entrées as well as fast-food or other restaurant choices for those hectic days when there is no time to prepare healthy meals.

Each menu section begins with simple menus that need little or no preparation and include convenience foods and restaurant selections, followed by menus that include easy-to-fix recipes for the main entrées and serving suggestions to round out each meal. The side-dishes recipe section includes recipes for dishes that are listed in several of the menus.

At the end of each menu, the food exchange numbers are listed to aid you in planning. As you will notice, each breakfast, lunch or dinner menu has a similar set of exchange amounts. This will make it simple for you to plan a day's worth of menus, knowing that no matter what meal combination you select for any one day, the exchanges for that day will fulfill the minimum requirements for a 1,400-calorie diet. You can increase the number of exchanges by adding planned snacks, double portions or additional side dishes to the meals.

> **Important Reminder:** Consult a physician before starting any weight-loss plan or making changes in your eating habits. The 1,400-calorie level is just a starting point for these menus and *not a recommended level for everyone*. A physician or a registered dietitian can help you determine your healthy weight and the calorie level needed to attain—and then maintain—your healthy weight.

HEALTHY LIVING

In addition to the delicious and convenient menus and recipes, this book provides a wealth of information related to making healthy eating choices. It includes information on a wide variety of topics, including tips on healthy shopping, the importance of eating breakfast, eating healthy while traveling and preventing serious health problems. Most of the articles were written by a physician and exercise physiologist, but a few were adapted from the *First Place Member's Guide*.

WEEKLY MEAL PLANNER

Week beginning_____ ending_____   Calorie level_____

Exchanges per day: Meats_____ Breads_____ Vegetables_____ Fruits_____ Milk_____ Fats_____

	Day 1:						Day 2:						Day 3:					
Breakfast																		
Exchanges	Mt	Br	Vg	Frt	Mk	Fat	Mt	Br	Vg	Frt	Mk	Fat	Mt	Br	Vg	Frt	Mk	Fat
Lunch																		
Exchanges	Mt	Br	Vg	Frt	Mk	Fat	Mt	Br	Vg	Frt	Mk	Fat	Mt	Br	Vg	Frt	Mk	Fat
Dinner																		
Exchanges	Mt	Br	Vg	Frt	Mk	Fat	Mt	Br	Vg	Frt	Mk	Fat	Mt	Br	Vg	Frt	Mk	Fat
Snacks																		
Exchanges	Mt	Br	Vg	Frt	Mk	Fat	Mt	Br	Vg	Frt	Mk	Fat	Mt	Br	Vg	Frt	Mk	Fat
Day's Total Exchanges																		

Key to abbreviations: Mt = meat; Br = breads; Vg = vegetables; Frt = fruit; Mk = milk; Fat = fats

Day 4:						Day 5:						Day 6:						Day 7:					
Mt	Br	Vg	Frt	Mk	Fat	Mt	Br	Vg	Frt	Mk	Fat	Mt	Br	Vg	Frt	Mk	Fat	Mt	Br	Vg	Frt	Mk	Fat
Mt	Br	Vg	Frt	Mk	Fat	Mt	Br	Vg	Frt	Mk	Fat	Mt	Br	Vg	Frt	Mk	Fat	Mt	Br	Vg	Frt	Mk	Fat
Mt	Br	Vg	Frt	Mk	Fat	Mt	Br	Vg	Frt	Mk	Fat	Mt	Br	Vg	Frt	Mk	Fat	Mt	Br	Vg	Frt	Mk	Fat
Mt	Br	Vg	Frt	Mk	Fat	Mt	Br	Vg	Frt	Mk	Fat	Mt	Br	Vg	Frt	Mk	Fat	Mt	Br	Vg	Frt	Mk	Fat

Sample
WEEKLY MEAL PLANNER

Week beginning __2/10__ ending __2/16__ Calorie level __1,400__

Exchanges per day: Meats __5-6__ Breads __6-7__ Vegetables __3-4__ Fruits __3-4__ Milk __2-3__ Fats __3-4__

	Day 1: *Sunday*						Day 2: *Monday*						Day 3: *Tuesday*					
Breakfast	p. 33 2 low-fat frozen waffles 1 tsp. reduced-calorie margarine 1 tsp. reduced calorie margarine ½ sm. mango 1 c. nonfat milk						p. 28 1 sl. cinn./raisin toast 1 tsp. reduced-calorie margarine ½ tsp. sugar ¾ c. plain nonfat yogurt ¾ c. blueberries						p. 29 1 Eng. muffin 1 tbsp. sugar-free syrup 1 c. strawberries 1 c. nonfat milk					
	Mt	Br	Vg	Frt	Mk	Fat	Mt	Br	Vg	Frt	Mk	Fat	Mt	Br	Vg	Frt	Mk	Fat
Exchanges		2		1	1	½		2		1	1	½		2		1	1	½
Lunch	p. 58 Chef salad 6 saltines						p. 00 Turkey Pepperoni and Veggie Pizza 1 sm. orange						p. 55 1 c. minestrone soup 6 saltines 1 c. salad 2 tbsp. low-fat ranch dressing ½ c. apple juice					
	Mt	Br	Vg	Frt	Mk	Fat	Mt	Br	Vg	Frt	Mk	Fat	Mt	Br	Vg	Frt	Mk	Fat
Exchanges	2	1	1	1		1	2	2	1½	1		1		1	2			1
Dinner	p. 00 Grilled Chicken w/ Corn Salsa Green beans Spinach salad Sm. dinner roll						p. 91 Smoked Turkey Quesadillas Creamy salsa						p. 84 Rosemary-Sage Steak Grilled vegetables Baked potato					
	Mt	Br	Vg	Frt	Mk	Fat	Mt	Br	Vg	Frt	Mk	Fat	Mt	Br	Vg	Frt	Mk	Fat
Exchanges	3	2	2			½	3	2	1	½		1	3	2	2			1
Snacks	¾ c. low-fat yogurt w/ ½ c. berries 1 med. banana						1 c. sugar-free, fat-free pudding 1 c. mixed raw veggies						1 sm. orange 2 oz. cheese					
	Mt	Br	Vg	Frt	Mk	Fat	Mt	Br	Vg	Frt	Mk	Fat	Mt	Br	Vg	Frt	Mk	Fat
Exchanges				2	1	1			1		1					1	1	
Day's Total Exchanges	5	5	3	4	2	3	5	6	3½	2½	2	2½	3	5	4	2	2	2½

Key to abbreviations: Mt = meat; Br = breads; Vg = vegetables; Frt = fruit; Mk = milk; Fat = fats

Day 4: Wednesday					
p. 25					
1 c. puffed-rice cereal					
½ med. banana					
1 c. nonfat milk					
Mt	Br	Vg	Frt	Mk	Fat
	1		1	1	
p. 43					
McDonald's Happy Meal (no mayo)					
1 c. green salad					
2 tbsp. low-fat dressing					
Mt	Br	Vg	Frt	Mk	Fat
2	3	1			2
p. 112					
Quick Baked Fish					
Brown rice					
Steamed broccoli					
Breadstick					
Mt	Br	Vg	Frt	Mk	Fat
3	2	1			1
1 sm. apple					
1 c. carrot sticks					
1 c. nonfat hot chocolate					
Mt	Br	Vg	Frt	Mk	Fat
		1	1	1	
5	6	3	2	2	3

Day 5: Thursday					
p. 28					
1 sm. bagel					
1 tsp. reduced-calorie margarine					
¾ c. raspberries					
1 c. nonfat milk					
Mt	Br	Vg	Frt	Mk	Fat
	2		1	1	½
p. 62					
Tuna-Salad Pita sandwich					
1 c. cucumber rounds					
1 c. carrot sticks					
15 grapes					
Mt	Br	Vg	Frt	Mk	Fat
2	2	1	1		1
p. 74					
Stouffer's Beef Macaroni Casserole					
Spinach salad w/mushrooms					
Peach					
Mt	Br	Vg	Frt	Mk	Fat
2	2	1	1		1
1 c. zucchini sticks					
½ c. nonfat cottage cheese w/ ½ c. pineapple					
Mt	Br	Vg	Frt	Mk	Fat
		1	1	1	
4	6	3	4	2	2 ½

Day 6: Friday					
p. 25					
¾ c. raisin bran					
1 slice diet wheat toast					
1 tsp. reduced-calorie margarine					
1 c. strawberries					
1 c. nonfat milk					
Mt	Br	Vg	Frt	Mk	Fat
	2		1	1	½
p. 64					
Stuffed Potato					
15 grapes					
Mt	Br	Vg	Frt	Mk	Fat
2	2	1	1		1
p. 76					
Salsa Beef and Turkey Loaf					
Garlic mashed potatoes					
Sautéed snap peas					
Mt	Br	Vg	Frt	Mk	Fat
3	2	1			2
½ c. tomato juice					
¾ c. flavored nonfat yogurt					
Mt	Br	Vg	Frt	Mk	Fat
		1	1	1	
5	6	4	3	3	3 ½

Day 7: Saturday					
p. 33					
2 frozen pancakes					
1 tbsp. sugar-free syrup					
½ med. grapefruit					
1 c. nonfat milk					
Mt	Br	Vg	Frt	Mk	Fat
	2		1	1	½
p. 54					
Turkey sandwich					
1 c. bell pepper strips					
1 c. nonfat coffee yogurt					
Mt	Br	Vg	Frt	Mk	Fat
2	1	1		1	½
Dinner Party at the Smiths					
Mt	Br	Vg	Frt	Mk	Fat
?	?	?	?	?	?
?					
Mt	Br	Vg	Frt	Mk	Fat
?	?	?	?	?	?
?	?	?	?	?	?

EATING HEALTHY, EATING RIGHT GROCERY LIST

Use this list to get you started and make copies so that you will have a list for each week.

BAKING GOODS

- [ ] _____ Baking soda
- [ ] _____ Baking powder
- [ ] _____ Cocoa
- [ ] _____ Cornstarch
- [ ] _____ Dried herbs
- [ ] _____ Nuts
- [ ] _____ Pepper
- [ ] _____ Raisins
- [ ] _____ Salt
- [ ] _____ Spices
- [ ] _____ Vanilla
- [ ] _____ _____
- [ ] _____ _____

BEVERAGES

- [ ] _____ Cocoa
- [ ] _____ Coffee
- [ ] _____ Fruit juice, 100%
- [ ] _____ Mineral water
- [ ] _____ Soft drinks, diet
- [ ] _____ Tea
- [ ] _____ _____
- [ ] _____ _____

BREADS

- [ ] _____ Bagels
- [ ] _____ Breads
- [ ] _____ Buns

- [ ] _____ English muffins
- [ ] _____ Rolls
- [ ] _____ _____
- [ ] _____ _____
- [ ] _____ _____
- [ ] _____ _____

CANNED GOODS

- [ ] _____ Applesauce
- [ ] _____ Beans
- [ ] _____ Chili
- [ ] _____ Fruit
- [ ] _____ Mushrooms
- [ ] _____ Soup
- [ ] _____ Spaghetti sauce
- [ ] _____ Stewed tomatoes
- [ ] _____ Tomato paste
- [ ] _____ Tomato sauce
- [ ] _____ Tuna/salmon
- [ ] _____ Vegetables
- [ ] _____ _____
- [ ] _____ _____
- [ ] _____ _____
- [ ] _____ _____

CONDIMENTS

- [ ] _____ All-fruit/jam/jelly
- [ ] _____ Honey
- [ ] _____ Ketchup
- [ ] _____ Low-fat mayonnaise
- [ ] _____ Mustard

- [ ] _____ Olive oil
- [ ] _____ Olives
- [ ] _____ Peanut butter
- [ ] _____ Pickles
- [ ] _____ Relish
- [ ] _____ Salad dressings
- [ ] _____ Salsa
- [ ] _____ Soy sauce
- [ ] _____ Syrup, diet
- [ ] _____ Vegetable oil
- [ ] _____ Vinegar

DAIRY

- [ ] _____ Cottage cheese
- [ ] _____ Cream cheese
- [ ] _____ Eggs/egg sub.
- [ ] _____ Low-fat sour cream
- [ ] _____ Milk, skim/1%
- [ ] _____ Other cheese
- [ ] _____ Parmesan cheese
- [ ] _____ Reduced-calorie margarine
- [ ] _____ Reduced-fat butter
- [ ] _____ Reduced-fat margarine
- [ ] _____ Yogurt (90-calorie)
- [ ] _____ _____
- [ ] _____ _____
- [ ] _____ _____

DRY GOODS

- ☐ _____ Beans/peas/lentils
- ☐ _____ Bread crumbs
- ☐ _____ Cereals
- ☐ _____ Cornmeal
- ☐ _____ Crackers
- ☐ _____ Flour
- ☐ _____ Oatmeal
- ☐ _____ Pancake mix
- ☐ _____ Pasta/noodles
- ☐ _____ Rice
- ☐ _____ Sugar/sugar sub.
- ☐ _____ Sugar-free pudding
- ☐ _____ Tortilla chips
- ☐ _____ _____
- ☐ _____ _____
- ☐ _____ _____
- ☐ _____ _____
- ☐ _____ _____

FROZEN FOODS

- ☐ _____ Frozen dinners
- ☐ _____ Frozen waffles
- ☐ _____ Light whipped topping
- ☐ _____ Light yogurt/ ice cream
- ☐ _____ Vegetables
- ☐ _____ _____
- ☐ _____ _____
- ☐ _____ _____
- ☐ _____ _____
- ☐ _____ _____

FRUIT

- ☐ _____ Apples
- ☐ _____ Bananas
- ☐ _____ Berries
- ☐ _____ Grapefruit
- ☐ _____ Grapes

- ☐ _____ Lemons
- ☐ _____ Limes
- ☐ _____ Melons
- ☐ _____ Oranges
- ☐ _____ Pears
- ☐ _____ _____
- ☐ _____ _____
- ☐ _____ _____
- ☐ _____ _____
- ☐ _____ _____

MEAT, FISH, POULTRY

- ☐ _____ Chicken
- ☐ _____ Deli Meat
- ☐ _____ Fish
- ☐ _____ Lean beef
- ☐ _____ Lean ground beef
- ☐ _____ Lean ham
- ☐ _____ Low-fat hot dogs
- ☐ _____ Low-fat sausage
- ☐ _____ Pork tenderloin
- ☐ _____ Shellfish
- ☐ _____ Turkey
- ☐ _____ Turkey bacon
- ☐ _____ _____
- ☐ _____ _____
- ☐ _____ _____
- ☐ _____ _____
- ☐ _____ _____

VEGETABLES

- ☐ _____ Broccoli
- ☐ _____ Cabbage
- ☐ _____ Carrots
- ☐ _____ Cauliflower
- ☐ _____ Celery
- ☐ _____ Cucumbers
- ☐ _____ Garlic
- ☐ _____ Lettuce

- ☐ _____ Mushrooms
- ☐ _____ Onions
- ☐ _____ Peppers
- ☐ _____ Potatoes
- ☐ _____ Radishes
- ☐ _____ Spinach
- ☐ _____ Tomatoes
- ☐ _____ _____
- ☐ _____ _____
- ☐ _____ _____
- ☐ _____ _____
- ☐ _____ _____
- ☐ _____ _____

MISCELLANEOUS

- ☐ _____
- ☐ _____
- ☐ _____
- ☐ _____
- ☐ _____
- ☐ _____
- ☐ _____
- ☐ _____
- ☐ _____
- ☐ _____
- ☐ _____
- ☐ _____
- ☐ _____
- ☐ _____
- ☐ _____

Conversion Chart for Equivalent Imperial and Metric Measurements

Liquid Measures

Fluid Ounces	U.S.	Imperial	Milliliters
	1 teaspoon	1 teaspoon	5
¼	2 teaspoons	1 dessert spoon	7
½	1 tablespoon	1 tablespoon	15
1	2 tablespoons	2 tablespoons	28
2	¼ cup	4 tablespoons	56
4	½ cup or ¼ pint		110
5		¼ pint or 1 gill	140
6	¾ cup		170
8	1 cup or ½ pint		225
9			250 or ¼ liter
10	1¼ cups	½ pint	280
12	1½ cups or ¾ pint		340
15		3/4 pint	420
16	2 cups or 1 pint		450
18	2¼ cups		500 or ½ liter
20	2½ cups	1 pint	560
24	3 cups or 1½ pints		675
25		1¼	700
30	3¾ cups	1½ pints	840
32	4 cups		900
36	4½ cups		1,000 or 1 liter
40	5 cups	2 pints or 1 quart	1120
48	6 cups or 3 pints		1350
50		2½ pints	1400

Solid Measures

U.S. and Imperial Measures		Metric Measures	
Ounces	**Pounds**	**Grams**	**Kilos**
1		28	
2		56	
3½		100	
4	¼	112	
5		140	
6		168	
8	½	225	
9		250	¼
12	¾	340	
16	1	450	
18		500	½
20	1¼	560	
24		675	
27		750	¾
32	2	900	
36	2¼	1,000	1
40	2½	1,100	
48	3	1,350	
54		1,500	1½
64	4	1,800	
72	4½	2,000	2
80	5	2,250	2¼
100	6	2,800	2¾

Oven Temperature Equivalents

Fahrenheit	Celsius	Gas Mark	Description
225	110	¼	Cool
250	130	½	
275	140	1	Very Slow
300	150	2	
325	170	3	Slow
350	180	4	Moderate
375	190	5	
400	200	6	Moderately Hot
425	220	7	Fairly Hot
450	230	8	Hot
475	240	9	Very Hot
500	250	10	Extremely Hot

BREAKFASTS

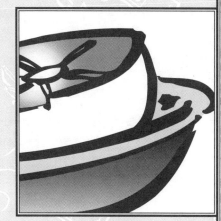

Note: Recipes for **boldfaced** items can be found in "Side Dishes" beginning on page 125.

Breakfast Menus

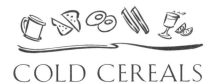

COLD CEREALS

1 c. bran-flakes cereal, with
  1 c. nonfat milk
½ medium papaya
Exchanges: 2 breads, 1 fruit, 1 milk

1 c. bran-flakes cereal, with
  2 tbsp. raisins and
  1 c. nonfat milk
Exchanges: 2 breads, 1 fruit, 1 milk

½ c. bran-flakes cereal, with
  1 tbsp. raisins and
  1 c. nonfat milk
1 slice whole-wheat bread, toasted and topped with
  1 tsp. all-fruit spread
Exchanges: 2 breads, ½ fruit, 1 milk

½ c. cornflakes cereal, with
  ½ c. sliced strawberries and
  1 c. nonfat milk
2 slices diet whole-wheat bread, toasted and topped with
  1 tbsp. fat-free cream cheese
Exchanges: ½ meat, 2 breads, ½ fruit, 1 milk

½ c. cornflakes cereal, with
  ½ medium banana, sliced, and
  1 c. nonfat milk
2 slices diet whole-wheat bread, toasted and topped with
  1 tsp. reduced-calorie margarine
Exchanges: 2 breads, 1 fruit, 1 milk, ½ fat

¾ c. cornflakes cereal, with
1 c. nonfat milk
½ small (2 oz.) bagel, toasted
1 c. mixed melon cubes
Exchanges: 2 breads, 1 fruit, 1 milk

1 c. fortified-flake cereal, with
1 c. nonfat milk
½ small mango
Exchanges: 2 breads, 1 fruit, 1 milk

1 c. fortified-flake cereal, with
1 small banana and
1 c. nonfat milk
Exchanges: 1½ breads, 1 fruit, 1 milk

1 c. Kellogg's Nutri-Grain
cereal, with
2 tbsp. raisins and
1 c. nonfat milk
Exchanges: 2 breads, 1 fruit, 1 milk

½ c. oat-bran cereal, with
½ medium banana and
1 c. nonfat milk
**Exchanges: 2 breads, 1 fruit, 1 milk,
½ fat**

1 c. puffed-rice cereal, with
½ medium banana, sliced, and
1 c. nonfat milk
Exchanges: 1 bread, 1 fruit, 1 milk

1½ c. puffed-rice cereal, with
1 c. fresh berries in season and
1 c. nonfat milk
Exchanges: 2 breads, 1 fruit, 1 milk

1½ c. puffed-wheat cereal, with
1 c. nonfat milk
1 large tangerine
Exchanges: 1 bread, 1 fruit, 1 milk

¾ c. raisin-bran cereal, with
1 c. sliced strawberries and
1 c. nonfat milk
1 slice diet wheat bread, toasted
and topped with
1 tsp. reduced-calorie margarine
**Exchanges: 2 breads, 1 fruit, 1 milk,
½ fat**

1 c. raisin-bran cereal, with
½ c. nonfat milk
6 oz. plain nonfat yogurt,
topped with
¼ c. pineapple chunks and
1 tsp. All-Bran cereal
Exchanges: 2 breads, 1 fruit, 1 milk

1 c. wheat-flakes cereal, with
1 medium peach, sliced, and
1 c. nonfat milk
Exchanges: 2 breads, 1 fruit, 1 milk

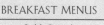

¾ c. Rice Chex cereal, with
   ½ medium banana and
   1 c. nonfat milk
½ English muffin, toasted and
   topped with
      ½ tsp. reduced-fat margarine
      and
      1 tsp. all-fruit spread
**Exchanges: 2 breads, 1 fruit, 1 milk,
¼ fat**

¾ c. Special K cereal, with
   1 small banana and
   1 c. nonfat milk
½ small (2 oz.) whole-wheat
   bagel, toasted and topped with
      1 tsp. low-fat peanut butter and
      1 tsp. all-fruit spread
**Exchanges: 2 breads, 1 fruit, 1 milk,
½ fat**

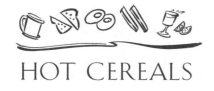

HOT CEREALS

½ c. cooked grits, topped with
  1 tsp. reduced-calorie margarine
1 slice diet whole-wheat bread,
  toasted and topped with
  1 tsp. all-fruit spread
1 small banana
1 c. nonfat milk
**Exchanges: 2 breads, 1 fruit, 1 milk,
½ fat**

½ c. cooked grits, topped with
  1 oz. 2% cheddar cheese,
  shredded
1 slice diet whole-wheat bread,
  toasted and topped with
  1 tsp. all-fruit spread
½ c. orange juice
**Exchanges: 1 meat, 2 breads, 1 fruit,
½ fat**

1 c. cooked oatmeal
½ grapefruit
1 c. nonfat milk
**Exchanges: 1½ breads, 1 fruit,
1 milk, ½ fat**

½ c. cooked oatmeal
1 small (1 oz.) low-fat bran muffin
1 small orange
1 c. nonfat milk
**Exchanges: 2 breads, 1 fruit, 1 milk,
½ fat**

1 pkg. instant oatmeal (no sugar
  added), topped with
  2 walnut halves, chopped
1 small banana
1 c. nonfat milk
**Exchanges: 2 breads, 1 fruit, 1 milk,
½ fat**

1 c. cooked oatmeal, topped with
  ¼ tsp. reduced-fat margarine,
  Dash cinnamon,
  Dash nutmeg and
  2 tbsp. raisins
1 c. nonfat milk
**Exchanges: 1½ breads, 1 fruit,
1 milk, ½ fat**

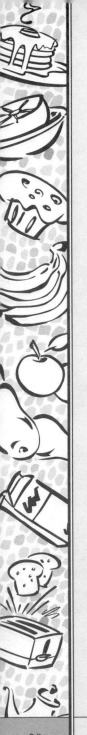

½ large (4 oz.) whole-wheat
  bagel, toasted and topped with
  1 tbsp. fat-free cream cheese
1 small orange
1 c. nonfat milk
Exchanges: ½ meat, 2 breads,
1 fruit, 1 milk

1 small (2 oz.) bagel, toasted and
  topped with
  1 tsp. reduced-calorie margarine
¾ c. raspberries
1 c. nonfat milk
Exchanges: 2 breads, 1 fruit, 1 milk,
½ fat

1 small (2 oz.) whole-wheat bagel,
  toasted and spread with
  1 tbsp. reduced-fat cream cheese
3 medium stewed prunes (or 2
  plums)
1 c. nonfat milk
Exchanges: 2 breads, 1 fruit, 1 milk,
½ fat

1 3-in. canned biscuit, topped with
  1 tsp. all-fruit spread
½ medium banana
1 c. nonfat milk
Exchanges: 1 bread, 1 fruit, 1 milk,
1 fat

2 slices cinnamon-raisin bread,
  toasted and topped with
  1 tsp. reduced-calorie margarine,
½ tsp. granulated sugar and
  Pinch cinnamon
¾ c. plain nonfat yogurt,
  combined with
  ¾ c. blueberries
Exchanges: 1 ½ breads, 1 fruit,
1 milk, ½ fat

2 slices diet sourdough bread,
  toasted and topped with
  1 tsp. reduced-calorie margarine
¾ c. blueberries
1 c. nonfat milk
Exchanges: 2 breads, 1 fruit, 1 milk,
½ fat

2 slices diet whole-wheat bread,
toasted and topped with
  1 tbsp. low-fat peanut butter
½ medium grapefruit
1 c. nonfat milk
**Exchanges: 1 meat, 1 bread, ½ fruit,
  1 milk, 1 fat**

1 small (2 oz.) diet blueberry muffin
½ c. cinnamon applesauce
1 c. nonfat milk
**Exchanges: 2 breads, 1 fruit, 1 milk,
  ½ fat**

1 small (2 oz.) diet bran muffin,
topped with
  1 tsp. reduced-calorie margarine
  and
  1 tsp. peach jam
½ medium banana
1 c. plain nonfat yogurt
**Exchanges: 2 breads, 1 fruit, 1 milk,
  ½ fat**

1 medium (3 oz.) diet bran muffin,
topped with
  1 tsp. low-fat peanut butter
¾ c. peach slices, canned in own
  juice, drained
1 c. nonfat milk
**Exchanges: 2 breads, 1 fruit, 1 milk,
  1 fat**

1 small (2 oz.) English muffin,
toasted and topped with
  1 tsp. reduced-fat margarine
½ medium grapefruit
1 c. nonfat milk
**Exchanges: 2 breads, 1 fruit, 1 milk,
  ½ fat**

1 small (2 oz.) whole-wheat
English muffin, split, toasted
and topped with
  1 tsp. reduced-calorie margarine
1 c. sliced strawberries
½ c. nonfat milk
**Exchanges: 2 breads, 1 fruit, 1 milk,
  ½ fat**

¾ c. artificially sweetened mixed-
berry nonfat yogurt, mixed with
¾ c. blackberries
1 small (2 oz.) bagel, topped with
  1 tsp. strawberry all-fruit spread
Exchanges: 2 breads, 1 fruit, 1 milk

1 English muffin, toasted and
topped with
  1 oz. slice Canadian bacon,
  sautéed, and
  1 slice tomato
1 small orange
**Exchanges: 1 meat, 2 breads, 1 fruit,
  ½ fat**

⅓ medium cantaloupe or honeydew
melon, topped with
  1 c. artificially sweetened
    pineapple-flavored nonfat
    yogurt and
  ¼ c. Grape Nuts cereal sprinkled
    on top
Exchanges: 1 ½ breads, 1 fruit, 1 milk

¼ medium cantaloupe, topped with
  1 c. plain nonfat yogurt,
  2 tbsp. raisins and
  1 tbsp. Grape Nuts cereal
    sprinkled on top
**Exchanges: ½ bread, 1 ½ fruits,
1 milk**

1 English muffin, toasted and
  topped with
  1 egg, poached
½ grapefruit
**Exchanges: 1 meat, 2 breads, 1 fruit,
½ fat**

¾ c. artificially sweetened fruit-
  flavored nonfat yogurt
1 small (2 oz.) sesame bagel,
  toasted and topped with
  2 tbsp. fat-free cream cheese
½ c. orange juice
**Exchanges: ½ meat, 2 breads, 1 fruit,
1 milk**

1 c. artificially sweetened fruit-
  flavored nonfat yogurt, mixed with
  1 medium-size fresh peach
    (or other fruit), sliced
1 medium (3 oz.) diet blueberry
  (or oat) muffin
**Exchanges: 2 breads, 1 fruit, 1 milk,
½ fat**

¾ c. artificially sweetened vanilla-
  flavored nonfat yogurt, mixed with
  ¾ c. blueberries
1 slice cinnamon-raisin bread,
  toasted and topped with
  1 tsp. reduced-fat margarine,
  ⅓ tsp. granulated sugar and a
  Pinch cinnamon
**Exchanges: 2 breads, 1 fruit, 1 milk,
½ fat**

1 c. plain (or artificially sweetened
  vanilla-flavored) nonfat yogurt,
  topped with
  3 tbsp. wheat germ (or 2 tbsp.
    Grape Nuts cereal)
1 slice whole-wheat (or 2 slices
  diet multigrain) bread, toasted
  and topped with
  2 tsp. all-fruit spread
6 oz. calcium-fortified orange juice
Exchanges: 2 breads, 1 fruit, 1 milk

1 c. plain nonfat yogurt,
topped with
  2 tbsp. Grape Nuts cereal
1 slice multigrain bread, toasted
  and topped with
  1 tsp. all-fruit spread
½ c. blueberries
**Exchanges: 2 breads, 1 fruit, 1 milk,
½ fat**

1 c. plain nonfat yogurt,
  topped with
  3 tbsp. wheat germ
1 slice whole-wheat (or 2 slices
  diet multigrain) bread, toasted
  and topped with
  2 tsp. all-fruit spread
6 oz. orange juice
Exchanges: 2 breads, 1 fruit, 1 milk

Fruit smoothie, made with
  1 c. nonfat milk,
  ½ medium banana and
  2 strawberries
2 slices multigrain bread,
  toasted and topped with
  2 tsp. all-fruit spread
(Note: See page 39 for some additional
great smoothie recipes!)
**Exchanges: 1 ½ breads, 1 milk,
1 fruit, ½ fat**

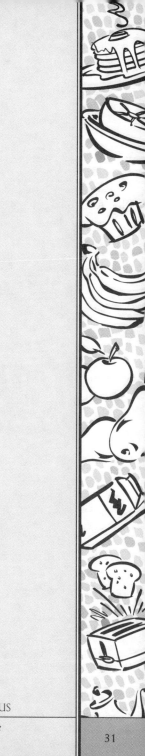

GRAB 'N' GO

Turkey bacon and egg sandwich,
  made with
  2 slices diet whole-wheat bread,
    toasted and topped with
  1 egg, cooked in a nonstick
    pan and
  1 strip turkey bacon, cooked
    crisp
1 medium apple
**Exchanges: 1 meat, 1 bread, 1 fruit,
    1 fat**

McDonald's Egg McMuffin
6 oz. orange juice
**Exchanges: 2 meats, 2 breads, 1 fruit,
    1 fat**

Breakfast pocket sandwich,
  made with
  1 6- or 7-in. whole-wheat pocket
    pita, heated and filled with
  ¼ c. 2% cottage cheese,
  ½ c. diced peaches, canned in
    own juice, and
  2 tsp. chopped walnuts
**Exchanges: 1 meat, 2 breads, 1 fruit,
    ½ fat**

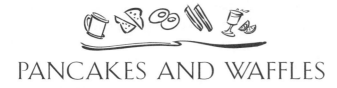

PANCAKES AND WAFFLES

2 frozen pancakes, heated and
  topped with
  1 tsp. reduced-calorie margarine
    and
  1 tbsp. sugar-free syrup
2-in. wedge honeydew melon
1 c. nonfat milk
Exchanges: 2 breads, 1 fruit, 1 milk,
  ½ fat

2 frozen pancakes, heated and
  topped with
  1 tbsp. sugar-free syrup
½ medium grapefruit
1 c. nonfat milk
Exchanges: 2 breads, 1 fruit, 1 milk,
  ½ fat

3 4-in. **Low-Fat Pancakes,**
  topped with
  1 tbsp. sugar-free syrup
1 c. sliced strawberries
1 c. nonfat milk
Exchanges: 2 breads, 1 fruit, 1 milk,
  ½ fat

3 4-in. **Low-Fat Pancakes,**
  topped with
  6 oz. plain nonfat yogurt,
    mixed with
    ½ c. chopped fresh
      strawberries and
    1 tsp. melted strawberry
      all-fruit spread
Exchanges: 2 breads, 1 fruit, 1 milk,
  ½ fat

2 low-fat frozen waffles, heated
  and topped with
  1 tsp. reduced-calorie margarine
    and
  1 tbsp. sugar-free syrup
½ small mango
1 c. nonfat milk
Exchanges: 2 breads, 1 fruit, 1 milk,
  ½ fat

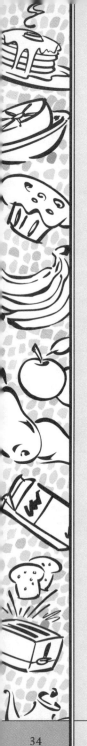

2 low-fat frozen waffles, toasted
  and topped with
    1 tsp. reduced-fat margarine and
    1 tbsp. sugar-free syrup
  1 c. honeydew melon balls
  1 c. nonfat milk
**Exchanges: 2 breads, 1 fruit, 1 milk,
½ fat**

2 low-fat frozen waffles, toasted
  and topped with
    ½ c. unsweetened applesauce,
      sweetened with
      1 pkg. artificial sweetener and
      2 tbsp. raisins
  1 c. nonfat milk
Exchanges: 2 breads, 2 fruits, 1 milk

2 low-fat frozen waffles, toasted
  and topped with
    2 tsp. strawberry all-fruit spread
  ½ c. sliced strawberries
  1 c. nonfat milk
**Exchanges: 2 breads, 1 fruit, 1 milk,
½ fat**

Breakfast Menus with Recipes

FRENCH TOAST, PANCAKES AND WAFFLES

RAISIN FRENCH TOAST

In a shallow bowl, combine egg substitute, vanilla and milk; add slices of bread, turning until egg mixture is absorbed. Spray a small nonstick skillet or griddle with nonstick cooking spray; preheat. Cook bread over medium heat 3 to 5 minutes, turning once, until golden brown on both sides.

Serve with 1 tablespoon sugar-free syrup, ½ cup grapefruit sections and ½ cup nonfat milk.
Exchanges: ½ meat, 2 breads, ½ fruit, ½ milk

Note: Recipes for **boldfaced** items can be found in "Side Dishes" beginning on page 125.

1 ½ slices cinnamon-raisin bread
¼ c. egg substitute
¼ tsp. vanilla flavoring
1 tbsp. nonfat milk
    Nonstick cooking spray

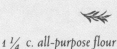

3 large eggs
1 c. plain low-fat yogurt
¼ c. unsweetened applesauce
½ tsp. vanilla extract
2 tbsp. sugar or Splenda® equivalent
   (don't use aspartame)
1 tsp. baking soda
¼ tsp. salt
1 c. all-purpose flour
1 c. blueberries*
   Nonstick cooking spray

*You may substitute an equal amount of raspberries, or chopped apples or pears for the blueberries. If you prefer not to use fruit, omit the fruit exchange.

1 ¼ c. all-purpose flour
½ pkg. Rapid Rise yeast
1 tbsp. sugar
½ tsp. salt
1 c. warm milk (105° F to 115° F)
2 large eggs
1 ½ tbsp. vegetable oil
1 tsp. vanilla extract

LOW-FAT PANCAKES

Separate 1 egg white and yolk into 2 large bowls. Add whites only from remaining 2 eggs into egg-white bowl; save extra yolks in refrigerator for another recipe. Add yogurt, applesauce, vanilla and sugar to egg-yolk bowl; stir with rubber spatula to mix. Stir in baking soda, salt and flour; blend well. Beat egg whites with electric mixer until stiff peaks form when beaters are lifted. Stir ⅓ of whites into batter until blended; gently fold in remaining whites until no white streaks remain.

Preheat griddle (or large skillet) over medium heat until a few drops of water flicked onto the surface skitter around and then disappear. Coat griddle with cooking spray. Pour G cup batter onto griddle; gently spreading to make a 4-inch pancake. If using fruit, quickly sprinkle on top; cook 2 minutes more or until bubbles appear on surface of pancake and underside is golden brown. Turn pancake over with broad metal spatula; cook 2 more minutes or until tops bounce back when touched. Makes 4 servings of 3 pancakes or 6 servings of 2 pancakes.

Exchanges: 3-pancake serving: ½ meat, 1½ breads, ½ fruit, ½ milk, ½ fat
2-pancake serving: ½ meat, 1½ breads

EASY WAFFLES

In large bowl, combine flour, yeast, sugar and salt. Add milk, eggs, vegetable oil and vanilla; stir just until blended. Cover and let rise in warm, draft-free place 45 minutes or until doubled in size (or cover and refrigerate overnight).

When batter is ready, bake in preheated waffle iron according to manufacturer's directions. Serve immediately with your favorite toppings such as sugar-free syrup, all-fruit preserves, fresh fruit and/or sweetened sour cream. Makes 4 servings of 2 4-inch waffles.

Exchanges (for waffles alone): 2 breads, 1 fat

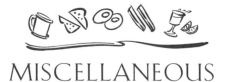

MISCELLANEOUS

BRUNCH CASSEROLE

Line bottom of 9x9-inch casserole dish with bread. Sauté sausage in nonstick skillet until done. Remove sausage and sauté mushrooms and onions until tender. Crumble sausage and combine with mushrooms and onion; sprinkle mixture on top of bread. Combine eggs, milk, salt, pepper and garlic; mix well and pour over sausage. Sprinkle with cheese; cover and refrigerate overnight. Set out for 15 minutes prior to baking. Bake at 350° F for 40 to 45 minutes. Serves 4.

    Serve each with ½ grapefruit.

Exchanges: 1½ meats, 1 bread, 1 fruit, ½ fat

4 slices wheat bread, crusts removed
2 oz. low-fat turkey sausage
¼ c. chopped mushrooms
1 tsp. chopped onion
3 eggs, beaten
1 c. nonfat milk
¼ tsp. salt
⅛ tsp. black pepper
⅛ tsp. granulated garlic
2 oz. low-fat cheddar cheese, shredded

BREAKFAST BURRITO

Scramble egg substitute, onion, bell pepper and salsa in skillet sprayed with nonstick cooking spray. Spoon ½ cooked mixture into each tortilla; roll into burrito.

    Serve with 1 small orange.

Exchanges: 1 meat, 2 breads, ½ vegetable, 1 fruit, ½ fat

2 6-in. low-fat flour tortillas
½ c. egg substitute
2 tbsp. chopped onion
2 tbsp. chopped bell pepper
2 tbsp. salsa
  Nonstick cooking spray

1 square (1½ in.) graham cracker,
   crumbled
8 oz. artificially sweetened vanilla-
   flavored nonfat yogurt, topped with
   2 tsp. chopped walnuts
½ c. sliced strawberries
   (or ½ c. blueberries)
3 tbsp. wheat germ (or 2 tbsp.
   bran cereal)

1 English muffin, split
2 slices tomato
¾-oz. slice fat-free ham, cut in half
2 slices pineapple
1 slice low-fat cheese, cut in half

½ c. egg substitute
¼ c. diced tomatoes
1 tsp. diced onion
1 tsp. diced bell pepper
   Nonstick cooking spray

BREAKFAST DELIGHT

Alternate ingredients in order by layering in parfait dish.
Exchanges: 2 breads, 1 fruit, 1 milk, 1 fat

OPEN-FACED HAWAIIAN BREAKFAST SANDWICH

Top muffin halves with slice each of tomato, ham, pineapple and cheese. Place in hot oven until cheese is melted.
Exchanges: 1 meat, 1½ breads, 1 fruit, ½ fat

SPANISH OMELETTE

Spray small frying pan with nonstick cooking spray. Combine ingredients and cook over medium heat until done.
  Serve with 1 slice diet whole-wheat toast and ½ cup fresh pineapple.
Exchanges: 1 meat, 1 bread, ½ vegetable, 1 fruit

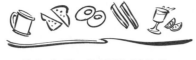

SMOOTHIES

CANTALOUPE-BANANA SMOOTHIE

Combine all ingredients in a blender and purée until smooth. Serves 2.
Exchanges: 2 fruits, ½ milk

1 c. *artificially sweetened vanilla-
flavored nonfat yogurt*
½ *small cantaloupe, peeled and cubed*
1 *medium banana, peeled and sliced*

PINEAPPLE-ORANGE-BANANA SMOOTHIE

Combine all ingredients in a blender and purée until smooth. Serves 2.
Exchanges: 1 fruit, ½ milk

¾ c. *artificially sweetened orange-
flavored nonfat yogurt*
1 *medium banana, peeled and sliced*
1 c. *pineapple-orange-banana juice*

POWER BREAKFAST SMOOTHIE

Combine all ingredients in a blender and purée until smooth. Serves 4.
Exchanges: ½ meat, ½ bread, 1 fruit, 1 fat

¾ c. *nonfat plain yogurt*
1 c. *orange juice*
¾ c. *peeled, diced apple*
1 *medium banana, frozen*
1 tsp. *vanilla extract*
3 tbsp. *smooth peanut butter*
2 tbsp. *wheat germ*

½ lb. silken tofu, drained
1 medium banana, peeled and sliced
2 c. unsweetened orange-pineapple juice, chilled
1 8-oz. can unsweetened, crushed pineapple, drained and chilled

1½ c. artificially sweetened vanilla-flavored nonfat yogurt
1 medium banana, peeled and sliced
¾ c. frozen peaches
1 10-oz. container whole frozen strawberries (no sugar added)
1 tbsp. orange juice concentrate

TROPICAL FRUIT SMOOTHIE

Combine all ingredients in a blender and purée until smooth. Serves 4.
Exchanges: ½ meat, 2 fruits

YOGURT SMOOTHIE

Combine all ingredients in a blender. Add enough ice to fill container; then purée until smooth. Serves 4.
Exchanges: 1½ fruits, ½ milk

LUNCHES

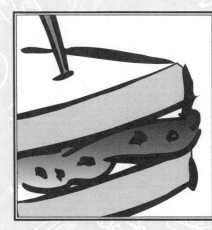

Note: Recipes for **boldfaced**
items can be found in
"Side Dishes" beginning
on page 125.

Lunch Menus

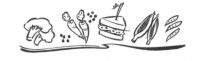

DINE IN/TAKE OUT

Arby's Roast Chicken Deluxe
sandwich (regular-sliced, no
mayonnaise)
1 c. green salad, tossed with
2 tbsp. low-fat dressing
½ c. celery sticks
1 apple
Exchanges: 2 meats, 2½ breads,
1 vegetable, 1 fruit, 1 fat

McDonald's chef salad, with
1 pkg. croutons and
1 pkg. low-fat dressing
1 c. carrot sticks
1 small low-fat frozen yogurt cup
1 small pear or apple
Exchanges: 2 meats, 2 breads,
2 vegetables, 1 fruit,
1 fat

Arby's Junior roast beef sandwich
1 c. green salad, tossed with
2 tbsp. low-fat dressing
1 small apple (or 1 medium banana)
Exchanges: 2 meats, 2 breads,
1 vegetable, 1 fruit, 1 fat

Arby's Light Roast Turkey
Deluxe sandwich
1 c. green salad, tossed with
2 tbsp. low-fat dressing
¼ c. peach slices, canned
in own juice
Exchanges: 2½ meats, 2 breads,
1 vegetable, 1 fruit, ½ fat

Boston Market Open-Faced
   Turkey Club sandwich
   (no cheese or sauce)
1 c. carrot sticks
2 tbsp. low-fat ranch dressing
1 c. fruit salad
Exchanges: 2 meats, 2 breads,
          1 vegetable, 1 fruit,
          ½ fat

Burger King kid's meal, with
   Small hamburger
   (no mayonnaise),
   Small French fries and
   Small diet soda
1 small apple
Exchanges: 1½ meats, 2½ breads,
          1 fruit, 2 fats

1 6-in. Subway Cold Cut Trio
   sandwich (no added fat or
   cheese), made with
   Lots of veggies
1 c. mixed berries
(Note: You may substitute 1 bag baked
potato chips for ½ of sandwich bread,
if desired.)
Exchanges: 2 meats, 2½ breads,
          1 vegetable, 1 fruit

Arby's Junior roast beef sandwich
1 c. cole slaw
1 c. mixed melon balls
Exchanges: 2 meats, 2 breads, 1 fruit,
          2 fats

McDonald's Happy Meal, with
   Small hamburger
   (no mayonnaise),
   Small French fries and
   Small diet soda
1 c. green salad, tossed with
   2 tbsp. low-fat dressing
Exchanges: 2 meats, 3 breads,
          1 vegetable, 2 fats

1 6-in. Subway club sandwich (no
   added fat or cheese), made with
   Lots of veggies
1 c. carrot sticks
2 tbsp. low-fat ranch dressing
15 red grapes
Exchanges: 2 meats, 3 breads,
          1 vegetable, 1 fruit, 1 fat

Taco Bell Burrito Supreme
1 c. green salad, with
   ¼ c. salsa and
   1 tbsp. low-fat sour cream
1 c. carrot sticks
½ c. fresh pineapple, cubed
Exchanges: 2 meats, 3 breads,
          1 vegetable, 1 fruit, 1½ fats

Taco Bell Light Chicken
    Burrito Supreme
1 c. gazpacho soup
1 small apple
Exchanges: 2 meats, 3 breads,
        1 vegetable, 1 fruit

Chick-fil-A Chargrilled
    Chicken sandwich
    Small carrot-and-raisin side salad
15 red grapes
Exchanges: 3 meats, 2 breads,
        1 vegetable, 1 fruit, 1 fat

1 c. Chinese take-out egg-drop soup
1 vegetable spring roll, with
    2 tsp. sweet-and-sour sauce
¾ c. steamed rice
1 medium peach
Exchanges: 1 meat, 2 breads,
        ½ vegetable, 1 fruit, 1 fat

FROZEN ENTRÉES

1 11-oz. frozen dinner entrée
1 c. fresh baby carrots
1 small apple
Exchanges: 2 meats, 2 breads,
        1 vegetable, 1 fruit, 1 fat

Healthy Choice Linguini
    with Shrimp
½ c. mixed-fruit salad
Exchanges: 1 meat, 2 breads,
        1 vegetable, 1 fruit

1 11-oz. Healthy Choice Pepper
    Steak entrée
1 c. green salad, tossed with
    2 tbsp. low-fat dressing
½ c. fruit salad
Exchanges: 2 meats, 2 breads,
        1 vegetable, 1 fruit

1 10- to 11-oz. frozen light dinner
    entrée (with 300 to 350 calories,
    fewer than 800 mg. sodium and
    fewer than 10 grams fat)
Spinach salad, made with
    2 c. spinach leaves,
    $\frac{1}{4}$ c. sliced mushrooms and
    2 tbsp. low-fat French dressing
15 grapes
Exchanges: 1 $\frac{1}{2}$ meats, 2 breads,
            1 vegetable, 1 fruit, $\frac{1}{2}$ fat

Stouffer's Lean Cuisine Hearty
    Portion Glazed Chicken with
    Vegetables and Rice
1 small banana
Exchanges: 2 meats, 2 $\frac{1}{2}$ breads,
            1 vegetable, 1 fruit, 1 fat

Stouffer's Lean Cuisine Fiesta
    Chicken
1 c. green salad, with
    $\frac{1}{2}$ c. diced tomatoes,
    $\frac{1}{4}$ c. diced cucumber and
    2 tbsp. low-fat dressing
1 small orange
Exchanges: 2 meats, 1 $\frac{1}{2}$ breads,
            1 $\frac{1}{2}$ vegetables, 1 fruit,
            $\frac{1}{2}$ fat

Stouffer's Lean Cuisine Chicken
    and Vegetables Vermicelli
2 c. green salad, tossed with
    2 tbsp. low-fat dressing
1 c. fresh citrus sections
Exchanges: 2 meats, 1 $\frac{1}{2}$ breads,
            1 vegetable, 1 fruit, $\frac{1}{2}$ fat

Stouffer's Lean Cuisine Lasagna
    with Meat Sauce
1 3-in. slice French bread, toasted
    Spinach salad, made with
    2 c. spinach leaves,
    $\frac{1}{4}$ c. sliced mushrooms and
    2 tbsp. low-fat French dressing
Exchanges: 2 meats, 2 breads,
            1 vegetable, 1 fat

Stouffer's Lean Cuisine Macaroni
    and Cheese
2 c. Caesar salad (salad kit),
    tossed with
    2 tbsp. low-fat Caesar dressing
1 orange
Exchanges: 1 $\frac{1}{2}$ meats, 2 breads,
            1 vegetable, 1 fruit, 1 fat

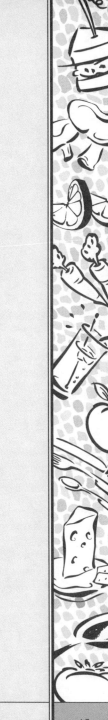

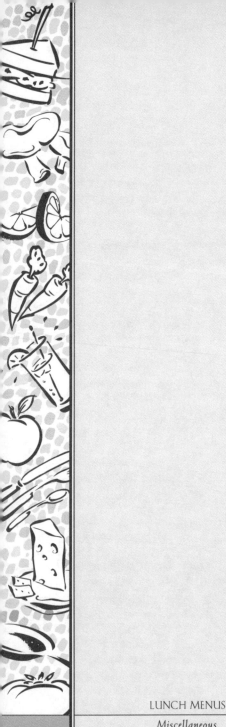

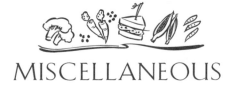

MISCELLANEOUS

1 6-oz. baked potato, topped with
   1 tsp. reduced-calorie margarine,
   ½ c. cooked chopped spinach
   and
   1 ½ oz. grated reduced-fat
   cheddar cheese
1 c. carrot sticks
1 c. celery sticks
**Exchanges: 1 ½ meats, 2 breads,
2 vegetables, 1 fat**

1 3-oz. baked sweet potato,
  topped with
   1 tsp. reduced-calorie margarine
   2 oz. cooked lean ham
1 c. combined steamed sliced
  zucchini and yellow squash
  Cucumber and tomato salad,
  made with
   1 c. sliced cucumber,
   1 c. sliced tomato and
   3 tsp. **Balsamic Vinaigrette**
1 small (1 oz.) dinner roll,
  topped with
   1 tsp. reduced-calorie margarine
**Exchanges: 2 meats, 2 breads,
2 vegetables, 1 fat**

1 6-oz. baked potato, topped with
   ½ c. cooked broccoli florets,
   ¼ c. sliced mushrooms,
   1 tbsp. chopped green onion,
   2 tbsp. shredded 2% cheddar
   cheese and
   1 tbsp. fat-free sour cream
1 small banana
**Exchanges: ½ meat, 2 breads,
1 vegetable, 1 fruit, ½ fat**

1 6-oz. baked sweet potato,
  topped with
   2 oz. cooked lean ham, diced
   1 tsp. reduced-fat margarine,
   1 tbsp. raisins and
   Dash cinnamon
1 c. asparagus spears, steamed
  and drizzled with
   1 tbsp. **Balsamic Vinaigrette**
**Exchanges: 2 meats, 2 breads,
2 vegetables, ½ fruit, 1 fat**

1 slice thin-crust cheese pizza
Mixed veggie salad, made with
   2 c. torn green leaf or
     romaine lettuce,
   ½ c. cooked artichoke hearts,
     chilled,
   2 oz. chickpeas, cooked and
     drained,
   ½ c. carrots,
   ½ c. zucchini sticks and
   2 tbsp. low-fat Italian dressing
1 small apple

Exchanges: 2 meats, 2 breads,
       2 vegetables, 1 fruit,
       1½ fats

2 oz. grilled boneless pork chop
⅔ c. cooked brown rice,
  topped with
   1 tsp. reduced-calorie
    margarine and
   ½ tsp. caraway seeds
1 c. steamed cabbage
2 c. green salad, tossed with
   1 tbsp. low-fat ranch dressing
1 small Granny Smith apple

Exchanges: 2 meats, 2 breads,
       2 vegetables, 1 fruit,
       1 fat

2 oz. roasted turkey
⅔ c. roasted new potatoes
1 c. steamed cauliflower
2 c. Bibb lettuce, tossed with
   ½ c. radishes,
   ¼ c. croutons and
   2 tbsp. balsamic vinegar
¾ c. blueberries

Exchanges: 2 meats, 2 breads,
       1 vegetable, 1 fruit

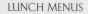

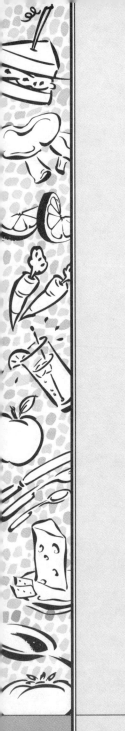

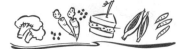

POULTRY AND SEAFOOD

2 oz. roasted boneless, skinless
chicken breast
⅔ c. cooked wide noodles, with
   1 tsp. reduced-calorie margarine
1 c. cooked sliced beets
Spinach salad, made with
   2 c. torn spinach leaves,
   ½ c. sliced mushrooms,
   ½ c. red onion,
   1 tbsp. imitation bacon bits
   and
   1 tbsp. fresh lemon juice
¾ c. plain nonfat yogurt,
  mixed with
   ½ c. peach slices, canned in
   own juice, drained
Exchanges: 2 meats, 2 breads,
    2 vegetables, 1 fruit,
    1 milk, ½ fat

2 oz. roasted boneless, skinless
chicken breast, cut into strips
1 slice diet French bread, toasted
  and topped with
   1 tsp. reduced-calorie
   margarine
½ c. cooked brown rice, with
   1 tsp. reduced-calorie margarine
½ c. each steamed whole green
  beans and julienne carrots,
  drizzled with
   ½ tsp. fresh lemon juice
2 c. mixed dark salad greens, with
  2 tbsp. low-fat blue-cheese
  dressing
1 small apple
Exchanges: 2 meats, 2 breads,
    1 vegetable, 1 fruit, 1 fat

2 oz. broiled boneless, skinless
chicken breast
Mixed bean salad, made with
1 c. cooked Italian green beans,
1 c. wax beans,
1 c. chickpeas, drained, and
1 tbsp. low-fat Italian dressing
2 small (1 oz.) breadsticks
½ tsp. reduced-fat margarine
1 small nectarine
Exchanges: **2 meats, 2 breads, 1 ½**
vegetables, 1 fruit, 1 fat

3 oz. broiled flounder
¾ c. new potatoes, boiled with
1 tsp. reduced-calorie
margarine and
1 tsp. minced fresh parsley
1 c. steamed zucchini slices
1 c. romaine lettuce, tossed with
2 tbsp. low-fat Thousand Island
dressing
1 small (1 oz.) breadstick
1 small orange
Exchanges: **2 meats, 2 breads,**
1 vegetable, 1 fruit, 1 fat

Shrimp cocktail, made on a bed of
4 romaine lettuce leaves,
topped with
4 oz. (about 12 medium)
cooked shrimp, peeled and
deveined, and
1 tbsp. cocktail sauce
3 slices (1 oz. total) cocktail
pumpernickel bread
1 serving **Pickled-Beet and**
Onion Salad
1 medium kiwi fruit
Exchanges: **2 meats, 1 bread,**
2 vegetables, 1 fruit, 1 fat

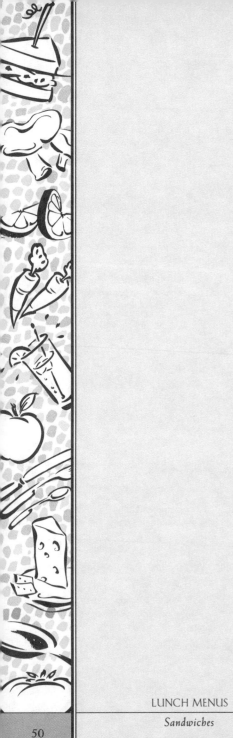

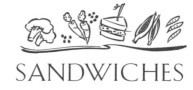

SANDWICHES

Veggie or garden burger,
made with
  ½ hamburger bun (or 1 whole
    diet bun),
  1 grilled or broiled veggie
    or garden patty (with at
    least 7 grams protein),
  1 tsp. prepared mustard,
  2 tomato slices,
  2 onion slices,
    Pickle slices and
  2 romaine lettuce leaves
1 oz. baked potato chips
1 kiwi, sliced
**Exchanges: 1 meat, 2 breads,
    ½ vegetable, 1 fruit**

BBQ pork sandwich, made with
  1 hamburger bun,
  2 oz. cooked pork tenderloin,
    sliced, and
  2 tsp. BBQ sauce
1 c. **Broccoli Slaw**
**Exchanges: 2 meats, 2 breads,
    1 vegetable, 1 fat**

Turkey burger, made with
  2 oz. hamburger roll,
  2 oz. grilled ground turkey patty,
  2½ tsp. **Russian Dressing,**
  1 slice nonfat processed
    American cheese,
  1 c. tomato,
  1 c. sliced Spanish onion and
  2 romaine lettuce leaves
Oven Fries
**Exchanges: 2½ meats, 3 breads,
    1 vegetable, 1 fat**

Hot dog, made with
  1 2-oz. frankfurter bread roll,
  1 2-oz. grilled fat-free
    frankfurter,
  1 tsp. pickle relish and
  1 tsp. prepared mustard
1 c. shredded mixed green and
  red cabbage, topped with
  1½ tsp. low-fat coleslaw dressing
1 c. carrot sticks
1 small apple
**Exchanges: 2 meats, 2 breads,
    2 vegetables, 1 fruit, ½ fat**

Cheese and veggie sandwich,
  made with
    2 slices diet whole-wheat bread,
    1-oz. slice reduced-fat Swiss
      cheese,
    ¼ c. roasted red bell-pepper
      strips, drained,
    ¼ c. alfalfa sprouts,
    ¼ c. spinach leaves and
    1 tbsp. low-fat Thousand
      Island dressing
1 8-oz. can ready-to-eat tomato soup
6 saltine crackers
1 c. broccoli florets
1 c. artificially sweetened raspberry-
  flavored nonfat yogurt, topped
  with
    ½ c. raspberries
Exchanges: 1 meat, 3 breads,
           1 vegetable, 1 fruit,
           1 milk, ½ fat

Peanut butter and banana
  sandwich, made with
    2 slices whole-wheat bread,
    1 tbsp. peanut butter and
    ½ medium banana, sliced
1 c. celery or carrot sticks
2 tbsp. low-fat ranch dressing
1 medium pear
Exchanges: 1 meat, 2 breads,
           1 vegetable, 1 fruit,
           1½ fats

Chicken sandwich, made with
    2 slices diet rye bread,
    2 oz. cooked boneless, skinless
      chicken breast, sliced,
    1 tbsp. fat-free Thousand
      Island dressing,
    2 tomato slices and
    ¼ c. shredded romaine lettuce
½ c. carrot sticks
½ c. zucchini sticks
2 tbsp. low-fat ranch dressing
1 small apple
Exchanges: 2 meats, 1 bread,
           1 vegetable, 1 fruit, ½ fat

Chicken salad sandwich,
  made with
    2 slices diet whole-wheat bread,
    2 oz. cooked boneless, skinless
      chicken breast, chopped,
    2 tsp. low-fat mayonnaise,
    ¼ c. chopped celery,
      Pinch freshly ground
      black pepper,
    2 slices tomato and
    2 romaine lettuce leaves
½ c. cucumber slices
½ c. carrot sticks
1 small banana
½ c. low-fat vanilla pudding
  (made with nonfat milk)
Exchanges: 2 meats, 1½ breads,
           1 vegetable, 1 fruit, ½ milk

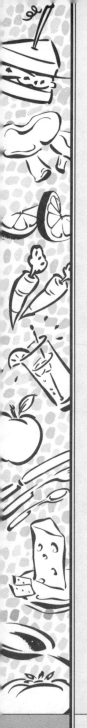

Roast beef sandwich, made with
   2 slices diet bread,
   1½ oz. cooked lean, boneless
      roast beef, thinly sliced,
   1 tbsp. low-fat Thousand
      Island dressing,
   2 slices tomato and
   2 romaine lettuce leaves
½ c. celery sticks
½ c. carrot sticks
1 c. sugar-free, white-grape-
   flavored gelatin, mixed with
   1 c. grapes
Exchanges: 1½ meats, 1 bread,
      1 vegetable, 1 fruit, ½ fat

Egg salad sandwich, made with
   2 slices diet rye bread,
   1 hard-boiled egg, minced,
   1 hard-boiled egg white,
      minced,
   2 tsp. low-fat mayonnaise,
   ¼ c. chopped celery and
   ¼ c. chopped red onion
1 c. carrot sticks
1 c. zucchini sticks
2 tbsp. low-fat ranch dressing
½ c. artificially sweetened
   chocolate-flavored nonfat
   frozen yogurt
Exchanges: 1½ meats, 2 breads,
      2 vegetables, 1 fat

Turkey sandwich, made with
   2 slices multigrain bread,
   2 oz. cooked turkey breast,
      sliced,
   1 tsp. low-fat mayonnaise,
   ½ tsp. prepared mustard
      (optional) and
      Pickle (optional)
Tossed salad, made with
   ¼ c. sliced tomato,
   ¼ c. sliced cucumber,
   ¼ c. sliced bell pepper,
   ¼ c. sliced carrots and
   2 tbsp. low-fat dressing
⅓ c. pineapple tidbits
Exchanges: 2 meats, 2 breads,
      1 vegetable, 1 fruit, 1 fat

Ham sandwich, made with
   1 English muffin, split and
      toasted,
   1 oz. cooked lean ham, sliced,
   1 tsp. low-fat mayonnaise,
   ½ tsp. prepared mustard,
   1 slice tomato and
   2 romaine lettuce leaves
1 c. broccoli florets, drizzled with
   1 tsp. low-fat dressing
Pear halves, canned in own juice,
drained and filled with
   ¼ c. 2% cottage cheese
Exchanges: 2 meats, 2 breads,
      1 vegetable, 1 fruit, 1 fat

Meatloaf sandwich, made with
   1 English muffin, split,
   2-oz. slice leftover
   Salsa Meatloaf,
   2 tomato slices and
   2 romaine lettuce leaves
½ c. artificially sweetened vanilla-
   flavored nonfat yogurt
1 c. mixed berries
**Exchanges: 1½ meats, 2 breads,
       1 fruit, ½ milk, ½ fat**

Turkey bagel sandwich, made with
   1 small (2 oz.) bagel,
   2 oz. cooked turkey, sliced,
   1 tsp. low-fat mayonnaise,
   2 tomato slices and
   2 romaine lettuce leaves
1 c. carrot sticks
1 apple
**Exchanges: 2 meats, 2 breads,
       1 vegetable, 1 fruit**

Sliced-egg sandwich, made with
   2 slices diet whole-wheat bread,
   1 hard-boiled egg, sliced,
   2 tsp. low-fat mayonnaise,
   ¼ c. watercress leaves and
   2 tomato slices
½ c. carrot sticks
½ c. celery sticks
3x2-in. watermelon wedge
**Exchanges: 1 meat, 1 bread,
       1 vegetable, 1 fruit, 1 fat**

Pastrami sandwich, made with
   2 slices diet rye bread,
   2 oz. cooked turkey pastrami,
   sliced,
   1 tsp. prepared spicy brown
   mustard,
   1 tsp. low-fat mayonnaise,
   2 tomato slices,
   ¼ c. alfalfa sprouts and
   2 romaine lettuce leaves
¼ c. **Summer Cole Slaw**
½ c. cucumber sticks
½ c. whole radishes
½ c. **Tropical Fruit Salad**
**Exchanges: 2 meats, 1 bread,
       1 vegetable, 1 fruit,
       1 fat**

Tuna sandwich, made with
   2 slices whole-wheat diet bread,
   1 4-oz. can water-packed tuna,
   drained,
   1 tbsp. low-fat mayonnaise,
   ½ tsp. pickle relish,
   2 tomato slices and
   2 romaine lettuce leaves
1 c. watermelon, diced
**Exchanges: 2 meats, 2 breads,
       1 fruit, ½ fat**

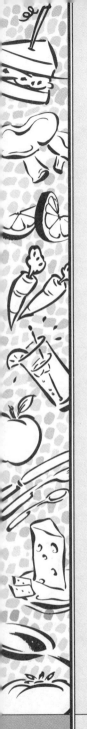

Honey-roasted turkey pocket
  sandwich, made with
  1 whole-wheat pita, split in
    half to form 2 pockets,
  1 tsp. low-fat mayonnaise,
  2 oz. honey-roasted turkey,
    thinly sliced,
  2 tomato slices and
  1 romaine lettuce leaf
½ c. red bell-pepper strips
½ c. zucchini sticks
1 small pear
**Exchanges: 2 meats, 2 breads,
      1 vegetable, 1 fruit, ½ fat**

Smoked-chicken sandwich,
  made with
  2 slices diet multigrain bread,
  2 oz. smoked boneless, skinless
    chicken breast, thinly sliced,
  2 tsp. low-fat mayonnaise,
  ¼ c. alfalfa sprouts and
  2 romaine lettuce leaves
Cucumber salad, made with
  ½ c. cucumber slices
  1 tsp. vegetable oil
  1 tsp. rice wine vinegar
    Pinch ground white pepper
1 c. artificially sweetened black
cherry nonfat yogurt
**Exchanges: 2 meats, 1 bread,
      1 vegetable, 1 milk**

Roast beef sandwich, made with
  1 6-in. whole-wheat pita, cut
    in half to form 2 pockets,
  2 oz. cooked lean, boneless
    roast beef, thinly sliced,
  1 tsp. low-fat mayonnaise,
  1 tsp. prepared mustard,
  2 tomato slices and
  1 romaine lettuce leaf
½ c. carrot sticks
½ c. cucumber sticks
**Exchanges: 2 meats, 2 breads,
      1 vegetable, ½ fat**

Turkey sandwich, made with
  2 slices diet rye bread,
  2 oz. roasted boneless, skinless
    turkey breast, sliced,
  1 tsp. low-fat mayonnaise,
  1 tsp. prepared mustard,
  ½ medium tomato, sliced, and
  ½ c. romaine or spinach leaves
1 c. mixed red and green bell-
  pepper strips
1 c. artificially sweetened coffee-
  flavored nonfat yogurt
**Exchanges: 2 meats, 1 bread,
      1 vegetable, 1 milk, ½ fat**

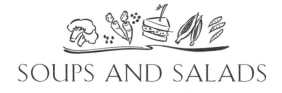

SOUPS AND SALADS

1 c. Campbell's Chunky
　　Minestrone Soup
6　saltine crackers
1 c. mixed dark salad greens, with
　　2 tomato slices,
　　½ c. baby carrots and
　　2 tbsp. low-fat ranch dressing
½ c. apple juice
Exchanges: 1 bread, 2 vegetables,
**　　　　　1 fat**

Turkey salad, made with
　　2 oz. cooked boneless, skinless
　　　　turkey breast, diced,
　　¼ c. chopped celery,
　　2 tbsp. chopped red onion,
　　2 tbsp. chopped spinach leaves,
　　1 tsp. fresh lemon juice and
　　2 tbsp. low-fat mayonnaise
½ c. each tomato and
　　cucumber slices, with
　　2 tsp. low-fat Italian dressing
2 rice cakes
1 pear
Exchanges: 2 meats, 2 breads,
**　　　　　2 vegetables, 1 fruit, 1 fat**

1 c. restaurant vegetable-beef soup
1 c. fresh fruit
Salad from salad bar, made with
　　2 c. mixed salad greens,
　　1 c. assorted vegetables and
　　2 tbsp. low-fat dressing
　　(**Note:** Go light on marinated
　　salads.)
Exchanges: 1 meat, 2 breads,
**　　　　　1 vegetable, 1 fruit, 1 fat**

Tuna-pasta salad, made with
　　½ c. cooked shell macaroni
　　1 4-oz. can water-packed tuna,
　　　　drained,
　　6 cherry tomatoes, halved,
　　¼ c. diced red onion and
　　1 tbsp. low-fat Italian dressing
½ c. carrot sticks
½ c. celery sticks
1 small (1 oz.) whole-wheat roll,
　　topped with
　　　　1 tsp. reduced-calorie margarine
1 medium peach
Exchanges: 2 meats, 2 breads,
**　　　　　1 vegetable, 1 fruit, 1 fat**

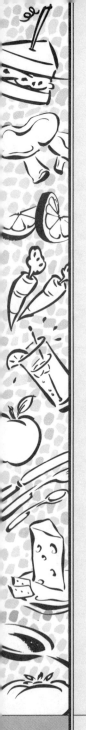

1 c. 90-calorie vegetable soup
20 oyster crackers
  Tossed salad, made with
    2 c. mixed dark green lettuce,
    ½ c. roasted red bell-pepper
      strips, chilled,
    ½ c. sliced celery,
    2 oz. reduced-fat cheddar
      cheese, diced and
    2 tbsp. low-fat Italian dressing
1 1-oz. slice Italian or French
  bread, topped with
    1 tsp. reduced-fat margarine
1 c. strawberries
Exchanges: 2 meats, 2½ breads,
**   2 vegetables, 1 fat**

  Green salad, made with
      Romaine lettuce or spinach
      leaves,
    ¼ c. sliced tomato,
    ¼ c. sliced cucumber,
    ¼ c. sliced bell pepper,
    ¼ c. sliced carrots and
    2 tbsp. low-fat dressing
2 small (1 oz.) breadsticks
½ c. **Marinara Sauce**, heated
1 oz. Parmesan cheese, grated
Exchanges: 1 meat, 1 bread,
**   1½ vegetables, ½ milk,**
**   1 fat**

1 8-oz. can beef barley soup
6 saltine crackers
  Dark green salad, with
    2 tbsp. low-fat dressing
2 slices pineapple, canned in
  own juice
Exchanges: 2 meats, 1 bread,
**   1 vegetable, 1 fruit, ½ fat**

1 c. Campbell's Chunky
  Manhattan-Style Clam Chowder
1 c. green salad, tossed with
    ½ c. cucumbers,
    ½ c. tomatoes and
    2 tbsp. low-fat dressing
Exchanges: 3 breads, 1 vegetable,
**   2 fats**

1 c. canned gazpacho soup
2 small (1 oz.) breadsticks,
  topped with
    2 oz. shredded low-fat Colby-
      Jack cheese, shredded
2 plums
Exchanges: 2 meats, 2 breads,
**   1 vegetable, 1 fat, 1 fruit**

1 c. canned chicken noodle soup

1 c. broccoli florets, with

    2 tbsp. low-fat ranch dressing

1 slice light Velveeta cheese

    (or 1 slice 2% cheese)

6 saltine crackers

2-in. wedge honeydew melon

Exchanges: 1 meat, 1 bread,

        1 vegetable, 1 fruit, 1 fat

Shrimp salad, made with

    2 oz. (about 6 medium) cooked

      shrimp, peeled, deveined and

      chopped,

    2 tsp. low-fat mayonnaise,

    ½ tsp. chili sauce,

    ½ tsp. fresh lemon juice and

    ½ tsp. sweet pickle relish

½ c. carrot sticks

½ c. celery sticks

2 c. watercress or romaine

  leaves, mixed with

    6 cherry tomatoes,

    1 c. sliced cucumber and

    2 tbsp. low-fat Italian dressing

1 small (2 oz.) bagel, toasted and

  topped with

    1 tsp. reduced-calorie

      margarine

15 grapes

Exchanges: 1 meat, 2 breads,

        2 vegetables, 1 fruit, 1 fat

Grilled chicken salad, made with

    2 oz. grilled boneless, skinless

      chicken breast, sliced,

    1 c. torn spinach leaves

    ½ medium tomato, sliced,

    ½ medium roasted bell pepper,

      sliced,

    ½ c. mandarin oranges,

    2 tsp. red wine vinegar,

    1 tsp. olive oil and

    Freshly ground pepper to taste

3 melba toasts

½ c. chocolate-flavored low-fat

  pudding

Exchanges: 2 meats, 1 bread,

        1 vegetable, 1 fruit,

        ½ milk, 1 fat

Tuna salad Nicoise, made with

    1 4-oz. can water-packed tuna,

      drained,

    2 c. shredded romaine lettuce,

    1 medium tomato, quartered,

    ½ c. cooked green beans,

    4 large black pitted olives and

    1 tbsp. low-fat Italian dressing

2 small (1 oz.) breadsticks

1 small banana

Exchanges: 2 meats, 2 breads,

        2 vegetables, 1 fruit, 1 fat

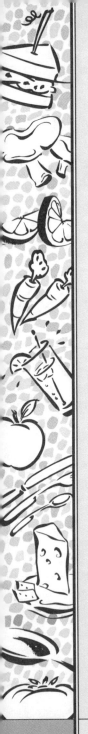

Chef salad, made with
    ¾ oz. cooked turkey, diced,
    ¾ oz. cooked ham, diced,
    1 ½ c. mixed salad greens
      (dark green),
    1 c. combined chopped
      broccoli, zucchini, carrots,
      onion, cauliflower and
      bell pepper,
    ¾ oz. reduced-fat Swiss
      cheese, diced,
    2 tbsp. reduced-fat dressing and
    ⅓ c. mandarin oranges
6 saltine crackers
Exchanges: 2 meats, 1 bread,
      1 vegetable, 1 fruit, 1 fat

Oriental seafood pasta salad,
    made with
    2 oz. (about 6 medium) cooked
      shrimp, peeled and deveined,
    ½ c. cooked rotini pasta,
    ½ c. bean sprouts,
    ½ c. sliced celery,
    ¼ c. cooked red kidney beans,
      drained,
    ½ c. mandarin oranges,
    1 tbsp. rice wine vinegar and
    ½ tsp. oriental sesame oil
½ pita bread, toasted
Exchanges: 1 meat, 3 breads,
      1 vegetable, 1 fruit, ½ fat

Spinach, bean and chicken salad,
    made with
    2 c. torn spinach leaves,
    ¼ c. cooked cannellini (white
      kidney beans), drained,
    2 oz. cooked boneless, skinless
      chicken breast, diced, and
    2 tbsp. low-fat Catalina-style
      dressing
½ c. carrot sticks
½ c. celery sticks
2 small (1 oz.) breadsticks
2 small plums
Exchanges: 2 meats, 2 breads,
      2 vegetables, 1 fruit,
      ½ fat

Spinach-mushroom salad,
    made with
    2 c. torn spinach leaves,
    ¼ c. sliced mushrooms,
    ¼ c. sliced red onion,
    1 hard-boiled egg, sliced,
    2 tsp. imitation bacon bits and
    2 tbsp. low-fat Italian dressing
½ c. celery sticks
½ c. carrot sticks
2 small (1 oz.) breadsticks
1 small peach
Exchanges: 1 meat, 2 breads,
      2 vegetables, 1 fruit, 1 fat

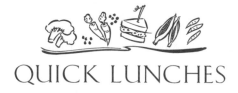

QUICK LUNCHES

2 oz. cooked lean ham, sliced thin
and wrapped around
　4 large cooked asparagus
　　spears and
½ c. cooked brown rice
1 pear
**Exchanges: 2 meats, 1½ breads,
　　1 vegetable, 1 fruit**

6 melba toasts
½ c. 2% cottage cheese
1 c. celery sticks
1　c. tomato juice
⅓ c. peach slices, canned in
　own juice, drained
**Exchanges: 2 meats, 1½ breads,
　　2 vegetables, 1 fruit**

6 saltine crackers, topped with
　2 oz. 2% cheddar cheese, sliced
1 small granola bar
4 canned apricot halves
**Exchanges: 2 meats, 2 breads, 1 fruit,
　　1 fat**

6 whole-wheat saltine crackers,
　topped with
　2 oz. 2% sharp cheddar cheese,
　　sliced
1 c. sliced cucumbers, marinated in
　2　tbsp. **Balsamic Vinaigrette**
1 orange
**Exchanges: 2 meats, 1 bread,
　　1 vegetable, 1 fruit, 1 fat**

6 whole-wheat saltine crackers
½ c. 2% cottage cheese
½ c. **Carrot Salad**
1 small low-fat granola bar
15 grapes
**Exchanges: 2 meats, 2 breads,
　　1 vegetable, 1 fruit, 1 fat**

4 graham-cracker squares, topped
　with
　1 tbsp. low-fat peanut butter
1 c. broccoli florets
1 apple, sliced
**Exchanges: 1 meat, 1 bread,
　　1 vegetable, 1 fruit, 1 fat**

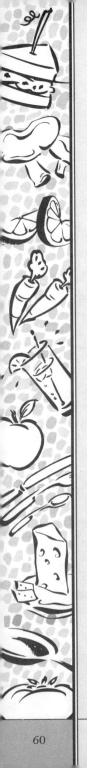

½ c. 2% cottage cheese, topped
  with
  ¼ c. chopped tomatoes,
  ¼ c. alfalfa sprouts and
  ½ tbsp. chopped scallions
  2 slices diet rye bread, toasted
    and topped with
    2 tsp. reduced-calorie margarine
1 c. mixed red and green bell-
  pepper strips
2 tbsp. low-fat ranch dressing
2 plums
1 4-oz. artificially sweetened
  chocolate-flavored nonfat frozen
  yogurt
Exchanges: 2 meats, 2 breads,
        1 vegetable, 1 fruit, 1 fat

1 small (2 oz.) sesame bagel,
  toasted and topped with
  1 tsp. reduced-calorie margarine
1 c. mixed carrot and celery
  sticks
½ c. 2% cottage cheese, mixed with
  ½ c. fresh pineapple chunks
Exchanges: 2 meats, 2 breads,
        1 vegetable, 1 fruit, 1 fat

Lunch Menus with Recipes

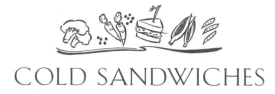

COLD SANDWICHES

Note: Recipes for **boldfaced** items can be found in "Side Dishes" beginning on page 125.

TUNA POCKET SANDWICH

In small bowl, combine tuna, mayonnaise and pickle relish. Fill each pita pocket with half of tuna salad; top each with half of romaine lettuce.

    Serve with ½ cup carrot sticks, 1 teaspoon low-fat ranch dressing and 1¼ cups watermelon.

Exchanges: 2 meats, 2 breads, 1 vegetable, 1 fruit, ½ fat

1   7-in. wheat pita, cut in half crosswise to form 2 pockets

1   4-oz. can water-packed tuna, drained

1   tbsp. low-fat mayonnaise

1   tsp. sweet pickle relish

½   c. shredded romaine lettuce

VEGGIE POCKET SANDWICH

Fill each pita pocket with ½ ounce cheese, 4 cucumber slices, 2 tomato slices and 1½ teaspoons dressing.

    Serve with 1 small apple.

Exchanges: 1 meat, 2 breads, 1 vegetable, 1 fruit, 1 fat

1   7-in. whole-wheat pita, cut in half crosswise to form 2 pockets

1   oz. 2% cheddar cheese, sliced

8   cucumber slices

4   tomato slices

½   tbsp. low-fat ranch dressing

1 7-in. whole-wheat pita, cut in half
   crosswise to form 2 pockets
1 4-oz. can water-packed tuna, drained
¼ c. chopped onion
¼ c. chopped celery
2 tsp. low-fat mayonnaise
¼ tsp. lemon-pepper seasoning
½ c. alfalfa sprouts

TUNA SALAD PITA SANDWICH

In small bowl, combine tuna, onion, celery, mayonnaise and lemon-pepper seasoning. Fill each pita pocket with half of tuna salad; top each with ¼ cup alfalfa sprouts.

   Serve with 1 cup cucumber rounds, 1 cup carrot sticks and 15 grapes.
Exchanges: 2 meats, 2 breads, 1 vegetable, 1 fruit, 1 fat

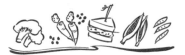

HOT OFF THE GRILL

OPEN-FACED REUBEN SANDWICH

2 slices diet rye bread
½ tbsp. low-fat Thousand Island
   dressing
1½ oz. lean corned beef, thinly sliced
½ c. sauerkraut, drained
½ oz. low-fat Swiss cheese, sliced
   Black pepper, freshly ground

Veggie Dip (*Combine ingredients ahead of time; mix well and refrigerate.)
  ¼ c. plain nonfat yogurt
  2 tbsp. prepared mustard

While broiler is preheating, lightly toast bread; spread each toast slice with 1½ teaspoons dressing. Place toast slices (spread side up) onto rack in broiler pan. Layer each slice with half each of corned beef, sauerkraut and cheese, in order. Sprinkle evenly with pepper to taste. Broil 4 inches from heat for 2 minutes or until cheese is melted and lightly browned.

   Serve with ½ cup carrot sticks, ½ cup cauliflower florets and ½ cup sugar-free, cherry-flavored gelatin mixed with fruit cocktail.
Exchanges: 2 meats, 2 breads, 1 vegetable, 1 fruit, 1 fat

GRILLED TURKEY AND CHEESE SANDWICH

Preheat skillet; coat with cooking spray. Spread mayonnaise and mustard on bread; layer with turkey and cheese. Grill sandwich over medium heat until bread is lightly browned on both sides and cheese is melted, turning occasionally. Combine tomato and cucumber in small bowl; drizzle with dressing prior to serving.

Serve with 1 ounce reduced-fat pretzels.

Exchanges: 2 meats, 2 breads, 1 vegetable, 1 fat

2 slices whole-wheat diet bread
1½-oz. slice cooked turkey breast
½-oz. slice Swiss cheese
1 tsp. low-fat mayonnaise
1 tsp. prepared mustard
1 medium tomato, quartered
½ cucumber, quartered
1 tbsp. **Balsamic Vinaigrette**
  Butter-flavored nonstick
  cooking spray

BROILED HAM AND CHEESE SANDWICH

Preheat broiler. Lightly toast bread. Layer ham, tomato and cheese on each slice of toasted bread; broil 4 inches from heat for 2 minutes or until cheese is melted and lightly browned.

Serve with 1⅓ cups **Mixed Bean Salad** and 1 small pear.

Exchanges: 2 meats, 1 bread, 2 vegetables, 1 fruit, 1 fat

2 slices diet whole-wheat bread
½ oz. cooked lean ham, thinly sliced
2 tomato slices
½ slice processed, nonfat American
  cheese
1 small pear

FRENCH-DIP ROAST BEEF SANDWICH

Cut bread loaf in half horizontally; then cut pieces in half vertically to make 4 pieces. Place 2 bread pieces, cut side up, on each of 2 plates. Top each with 1 ounce of roast beef and ¼ cup broth. Cover each plate with plastic wrap; microwave for 30 to 45 seconds, until hot. Serves 2.

Serve each with 1 cup broccoli florets topped with 2 tablespoons low-fat ranch dressing, and 1 cup strawberries.

Exchanges: 2 meats, 2 breads, 1 vegetable, 1 fruit, 1 fat

1 4-oz. loaf French bread
4 oz. cooked, lean boneless roast beef,
  thinly sliced
1 c. low-sodium beef broth, heated

2 slices whole-grain bread, toasted
1 oz. canned white chicken meat,
    drained and combined with
2 tsp. low-fat mayonnaise
1 oz. low-fat mozzarella cheese,
    shredded

CHICKEN PATTY MELT

Preheat broiler. In small bowl, combine chicken and mayonnaise; set aside. Place bread onto rack in broiler pan; top with chicken mixture and cheese. Broil open-faced until cheese is melted.

Serve with 1 cup celery sticks with 1 tablespoon fat-free ranch dressing, and 1 medium apple.

Exchanges: 2 meats, 2 breads, 1 vegetable, 1 fruit, 1 fat

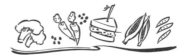

MISCELLANEOUS

1 6-oz. baked potato
1 oz. low-fat cheddar cheese, shredded
1 oz. cooked turkey bacon, crumbled
¼ c. cooked broccoli florets
¼ c. diced tomato
1 tbsp. diced green onion
¼ c. sliced mushrooms
1 tbsp. fat-free sour cream
1 tsp. reduced-fat margarine

STUFFED POTATO

Cut potato in half lengthwise. Scoop out potato "meat" from skins into small bowl; set skins aside. Combine cheese, bacon, broccoli, tomato, green onion, mushrooms, sour cream and margarine with potato meat; mix well. Refill shells with mixture; cover with plastic wrap and place in microwave-safe dish. Microwave until hot.

Serve with 15 grapes.

Exchanges: 2 meats, 2 breads, 1 vegetable, 1 fruit, 1 fat

CHEESE QUESADILLA

Place one tortilla in preheated skillet sprayed with cooking spray. Add half of cheese to one side of tortilla; fold over top. Cook over medium heat 2 minutes each side or until brown; repeat for second tortilla.

    Serve with salsa, sour cream and 4 celery sticks with 1 tablespoon reduced-fat ranch dressing.

Exchanges: 2 meats, 2 breads, 1 ½ vegetables, 1 fat

2 6-in. low-fat flour tortillas
2 oz. 2% cheddar cheese, sliced
½ c. salsa
¼ c. fat-free sour cream
    Nonstick cooking spray

VEGGIE CHEESE QUESADILLA

Place one tortilla in preheated skillet sprayed with cooking spray. In order, add cheese, broccoli and mushrooms to tortilla; cover with second tortilla and brown each side. Remove from pan and let sit 1 minute. Slice and serve with sour cream and salsa.

    Serve with 1 tablespoon low-fat sour cream, ¼ cup salsa, 1 cup carrot sticks and ½ cup sliced peaches in own juice.

Exchanges: 2 meats, 2 breads, 2 vegetables, 1 fruit, 1 fat

2 6-in. low-fat flour tortillas
2 oz. low-fat Colby-Jack cheese, grated
½ c. cooked broccoli florets
¼ c. sliced mushrooms
    Nonstick cooking spray

BBQ FRANK AND BEANS

Combine all ingredients in microwave-safe bowl. Microwave on high for 2 to 3 minutes or until hot.

    Serve with 1 cup peeled, sliced cucumber tossed with 1 tablespoon low-fat Italian dressing, and 1 cup cantaloupe cubes.

Exchanges: 2 meats, 2 breads, 1 vegetable, 1 fruit, 1 fat

1 cooked low-fat all-beef frank, diced
1 c. baked beans, drained
1 tbsp. prepared BBQ sauce

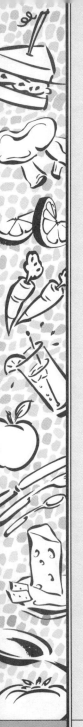

1 6-in. flat pita bread

¼ c. prepared chunky-style spaghetti sauce

8 turkey pepperoni slices

¼ c. shredded carrots

¼ c. cooked broccoli florets

¼ c. diced tomatoes

1 oz. low-fat mozzarella cheese, shredded

---

1 English muffin, toasted

2 c. frozen, chopped broccoli

½ c. low-sodium chicken broth

½ c. nonfat milk

2 hard-boiled egg whites, chopped

1 hard-boiled egg with yolk, chopped

1 tbsp. finely chopped celery

2 tsp. low-fat mayonnaise

Salt and pepper to taste

---

1 ½ oz. cooked chicken, shredded

¼ c. diced onion

¼ c. diced bell pepper

¼ c. salsa

1 tbsp. fat-free sour cream

1 10-in. low-fat flour tortilla

¼ oz. Colby-Jack cheese, shredded

Nonstick cooking spray

TURKEY PEPPERONI AND VEGGIE PIZZA

Preheat oven to 450° F. Place pita bread on cookie sheet; spread spaghetti sauce over bread. Layer with remaining ingredients, finishing with cheese. Bake 8 to 10 minutes or until cheese is melted.

Serve with 1 small orange.

Exchanges: 2 meats, 2 breads, 1 ½ vegetables, 1 fruit, 1 fat

EGG SALAD MUFFIN WITH BROCCOLI BISQUE

Combine broccoli, chicken broth and milk in food processor; purée until smooth. In small bowl, combine eggs, celery, mayonnaise, salt and pepper. Mix well and set aside. Transfer broccoli mixture to saucepan and cook over medium heat until hot. While heating bisque, scoop egg mixture onto toasted English muffin.

Serve with 1 small apple.

Exchanges: 2 meats, 2 breads, 2 vegetables, 1 fruit, 1 fat

QUICK CHICKEN FAJITA

In skillet coated with cooking spray, sauté onion and bell pepper for 1 minute; add chicken and heat thoroughly. In small bowl, combine salsa and sour cream; mix well. Fill tortilla with chicken; top with cheese. Heat in microwave, if desired, and serve with creamy salsa.

Serve with 1 cup canned mixed tropical fruit.

Exchanges: 2 meats, 2 breads, 1 ½ vegetables, 1 fruit, 1 fat

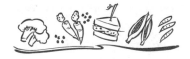

SALADS

BEAN AND SALSA SALAD

In small bowl, combine kidney beans, cheese, onion, salsa and lime juice.
Line plate with spinach leaves; top with bean mixture, sour cream and cilantro.
    Serve with 1 ounce nonfat tortilla chips and ½ small mango.
Exchanges: 2 meats, 2 breads, 1 vegetable, 1 fruit, 1 fat

WALDORF SALAD WITH CHEESE

In small bowl, combine apple, celery, cheese and mayonnaise. Top cabbage
with mixture.
    Serve with three 2½-inch square graham crackers.
Exchanges: 2 meats, 2 breads, 1 vegetable, 1 fruit, 1 fat

½ c. cooked red kidney beans, drained
1½ oz. Pepper-Jack cheese, shredded
½ c. finely chopped red onion
¼ c. salsa
1 tsp. fresh lime juice
1 c. spinach leaves, tightly packed
2 tbsp. fat-free sour cream
1 tsp. minced fresh cilantro

1 small apple, cored and diced
½ c. chopped celery
2 oz. low-fat cheddar cheese, grated
2 tsp. low-fat mayonnaise
2 c. shredded red cabbage

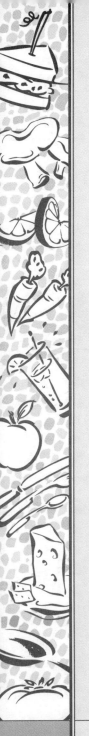

FRUITED CHICKEN SALAD

8 oz. cooked chicken breast, diced
¼ c. diced celery
1 small apple, diced
½ c. seedless red grapes, halved
½ c. mandarin orange slices
2 walnut halves, chopped
⅓ c. low-fat mayonnaise
Mixed lettuce leaves
4 tomatoes, quartered

Combine chicken, celery, apple, grapes, oranges, walnuts and mayonnaise. Chill and serve on bed of lettuce with tomatoes as garnish. Serves 4.

Serve each with 8 whole-wheat crackers.

Exchanges: 2 meats, 1 breads, 1 vegetable, 1 fruit, 1 ½ fats

SHRIMP AND MACARONI SALAD

6 oz. uncooked macaroni
½ lb. frozen, cooked salad shrimp, thawed
¼ c. chopped red onion
1 c. diced red or green bell pepper
1 c. diced celery
1 medium tomato, diced
1 c. diced fresh pineapple
⅓ c. low-fat mayonnaise
¼ c. balsamic vinegar
1 tbsp. Dijon mustard
⅛ tsp. leaf basil
¼ tsp. black pepper

Cook macaroni according to package directions, omitting salt and fat; drain and set aside to cool. In medium bowl, combine shrimp, onion, bell pepper, celery, tomato, pineapple, mayonnaise, vinegar, mustard, basil and pepper. Add pasta; toss to coat. Chill before serving. Serves 4.

Serve each over 2 romaine-lettuce or spinach leaves.

Exchanges: 1 meat, 2 breads, 1 vegetable, ½ fruit, 1 fat

PASTA SALAD

Cook pasta according to package directions, omitting salt and fat; drain and set aside to cool. In small bowl, combine mayonnaise, mustard, vinegar, basil and black pepper; mix well. In large bowl, combine pasta, meat, onion, bell pepper, celery, tomato, cheese and dressing; toss and chill before serving. Serves 4.

Serve with ⅓ sliced cantaloupe.

Exchanges: **2 meats, 2 breads, 1½ vegetables, 1 fruit, 1 fat**

6 oz. uncooked rotini pasta

4 oz. cooked boneless, skinless chicken or turkey, diced

¼ c. chopped onion

1 c. sliced red bell pepper

1 c. sliced celery

1 c. cherry-tomato halves

4 oz. feta or blue cheese, crumbled

Dijon Dressing

⅓ c. low-fat mayonnaise

1 tbsp. Dijon mustard

¼ c. balsamic vinegar

⅛ tsp. leaf basil

¼ tsp. black pepper

CONFETTI SALAD

In large bowl, combine chicken, rice, bell peppers, carrots, corn, green onions, thyme, cheese and tomatoes; chill. Toss with dressing prior to serving. Serves 4.

Serve each with 1 small banana.

Exchanges: **1½ meats, 2 breads, 1½ vegetables, 1 fruit, 1 fat**

4 oz. cooked boneless, skinless chicken breast, diced

2 c. cooked brown rice

½ c. diced green bell pepper

½ c. diced red bell pepper

½ c. diced carrots

1 17-oz. can whole kernel corn, drained

4 green onions, chopped

1 tsp. dried thyme

2 oz. 2% cheddar cheese, shredded

½ c. cherry-tomato halves

⅓ c. low-fat Italian dressing

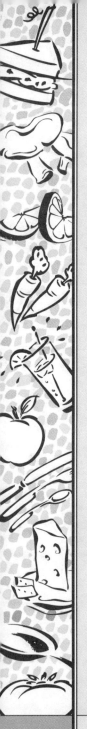

2 c. cubed cooked chicken

6 c. packed fresh spinach, washed and
   torn into bite-size pieces

2 oranges, peeled and cut into chunks

2 c. sliced fresh strawberries

Orange Poppy Seed Dressing
(*Combine ingredients ahead of time; mix
well and refrigerate.)

2 tbsp. red wine vinegar

3 tbsp. orange juice

1 ½ tbsp. canola oil

¼ tsp. dry mustard

¼ tsp. poppy seeds

12 oz. boneless, skinless chicken breasts

2 tsp. mild or hot chili powder

2 tsp. onion powder

1 tsp. garlic powder

1 tsp. paprika

8 c. torn romaine lettuce leaves

2 medium tomatoes, each sliced into
   8 wedges

1 c. cooked corn

2 thin red-onion slices, separated
   into rings

2 tbsp. low-fat ranch dressing

CHICKEN AND SPINACH SALAD

In large bowl, combine chicken, spinach, oranges and strawberries. Pour chilled dressing onto salad and toss just before serving. Serves 4.

Serve each with 6 slices melba toast.

Exchanges: 2 meats, 1 ½ breads, 1 vegetable, 1 fruit, 1 fat

BBQ CHICKEN SALAD

Preheat oven to 350° F. In small bowl, combine chili powder, onion powder, garlic powder and paprika; rub evenly over both sides of chicken breasts. Place chicken onto large sheet of foil; wrap tightly, crimping edges to seal. Place foil packet onto baking sheet; bake 8 to 10 minutes. Carefully open packet; bake 6 to 8 minutes more or until chicken is cooked through and juices run clear when pierced with fork. Set aside to cool.

While chicken is cooling, line large bowl with lettuce; top with tomatoes, corn and onion slices. Shred cooled chicken with fork; add to lettuce mixture. Drizzle evenly with dressing. Serves 4.

Serve with 1 cup broccoli florets, a 1-ounce whole-wheat roll with 1 teaspoon reduced-calorie margarine, and 1 medium peach.

Exchanges: 2 meats, 2 breads, 1 vegetable, 1 fruit, ½ fat

DINNERS

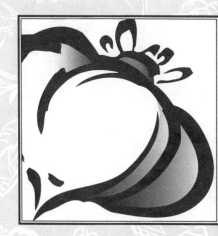

Note: Recipes for **boldfaced** items can be found in "Side Dishes" beginning on page 125.

Dinner Menus

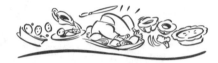

DINE IN/TAKE OUT

Captain D's or Long John Silver's
baked fish dinner, with
½ c. rice and
½ c. vegetables and
2 hush puppies or 1 small
(1 oz.) breadstick
**Exchanges: 3 meats, 2 breads,
1 vegetable, 1 fat**

1 fresh-roasted whole chicken
from your favorite store (remove
skin before eating) Serves 4.
Serve each with ½ cup mashed potatoes, 1 cup Italian green beans and a
1-ounce dinner roll with 1 teaspoon
reduced-fat margarine.
**Exchanges: 3 meats, 2 breads,
1 vegetable, 1 fat**

Seafood restaurant broiled or grilled
seafood entrée (lunch-sized
portion, sauce on the side),
with
½ c. rice and
½ c. steamed or
grilled vegetables
2 c. salad, with
2 tbsp. low-fat dressing on
the side
**Exchanges: 3 meats, 2 breads,
2 vegetables, 2 fats**

2 slices Pizza Hut Super Supreme
thin-crust pizza
2 c. salad, tossed with
2 tbsp. low-fat dressing
1 apple
**Exchanges: 3 meats, 3 breads,
2 vegetables, 1 fruit,
2 fats**

1 Taco Bell chicken fajita
3 tbsp. salsa
1 tsp. reduced-fat sour cream
1 c. mixed salad, tossed with
  2 tbsp. low-fat dressing
1 medium apple
Exchanges: **2 meats, 3 breads,**
          1 vegetable, 1 fruit,
          2 fats

2 slices Pizza Hut Supreme
  thin-crust pizza
1 c. salad, tossed with
  2 tbsp. low-fat dressing
1 c. sliced peaches, canned in
  own juice, drained
Exchanges: **3 meats, 3 breads,**
          1 vegetable, 1 fruit,
          2 fats

1 6 to 8-oz. steakhouse or restaurant
  chicken-vegetable kabob
1 stuffed potato (toppings on the
  side) *or* $\frac{1}{2}$ c. rice
$\frac{1}{2}$ c. vegetables
1 c. green salad, tossed with
  2 tbsp. low-fat dressing
Exchanges: **3 meats, 2 breads,**
          1 $\frac{1}{2}$ vegetables, 1 fat

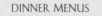

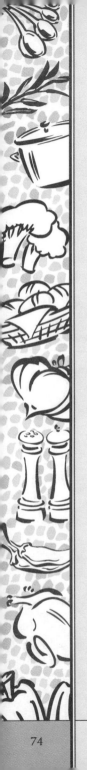

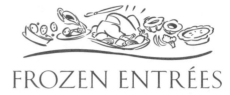

FROZEN ENTRÉES

1 10- to 11-oz. frozen dinner entrée
1 c. mixed-veggie salad, tossed with
  2 tbsp. low-fat dressing
1 frozen 100% juice bar
**Exchanges: 1½ meats, 2 breads,
      1 vegetable, 1 fruit,
      ½ fat**

1 Healthy Choice Glazed Chicken
2 c. salad, tossed with
  2 tbsp. low-fat dressing
1 small (1 oz.) dinner roll,
  topped with
    1 tsp. reduced-fat margarine
¾ c. fresh berries, topped with
  1 tbsp. nondairy whipped topping
**Exchanges: 2 meats, 2 breads,
      1 vegetable, 1 fruit, 1 fat**

1 Healthy Choice Chicken
  and Pasta Divan
2 c. salad, tossed with
  2 tbsp. low-fat dressing
½ c. fruit salad
**Exchanges: 2 meats, 2½ breads,
      1 vegetable, 1 fruit**

1 Stouffer's Beef Macaroni
  Casserole
Spinach Salad, made with
  2 c. torn spinach leaves,
    Mushrooms, to taste, and
  2 tbsp. low-fat dressing
1 peach
**Exchanges: 2 meats, 2 breads,
      1 vegetable, 1 fruit, 1 fat**

1 10- to 11-oz. frozen dinner
  entrée with meat
Salad, made with
  2 c. torn spinach leaves,
  ⅓ c. mandarin oranges and
    1 tbsp. low-fat sweet-and-
    sour dressing
1 small (1 oz.) breadstick,
  topped with
    1 tsp. reduced-fat margarine
**Exchanges: 2 meats, 2 breads,
      1 vegetable, ½ fruit,
      1 fat**

Dinner Menus with Recipes

Note: Recipes for **boldfaced** items can be found in "Side Dishes" beginning on page 125.

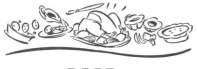

BEEF

BBQ BEEF AND NOODLES

Bring water to a boil. Place noodles in heat-resistant mixing bowl; cover with boiling water. Set aside for 20 minutes; then drain. In nonstick skillet, melt margarine over medium heat. Add onion; sauté 5 minutes or until soft. Add beef and mushrooms to skillet; increase heat to high and cook for 5 additional minutes, stirring constantly. Add water; reduce heat to low and continue cooking another 10 minutes.

While meat is cooking, mix together egg yolks, BBQ sauce and sherry. Scoop several spoonfuls of the meat mixture into bowl of egg mixture. Turn contents of bowl into skillet; heat gently while stirring. Serve over noodles. Serves 4.

Serve each with 2 cups spinach salad topped with ¼ cup croutons and 2 tablespoons low-fat dressing.

Exchanges: 3 meats, 2 breads, 2 vegetables, 2 fats

1 lb. leanest ground beef

4 oz. uncooked fine egg noodles

¾ c. water

2 tbsp. reduced-fat margarine

¾ c. diced onion

1 lb. mushrooms, sliced

2 egg yolks

3 tbsp. BBQ sauce

2 tbsp. cooking sherry

1 lb. lean (15% or less fat) ground beef
1 egg
2 tbsp. finely chopped green pepper
⅓ c. finely chopped onion
1 tsp. salt
2 slices bread, finely cubed
½ tsp. dry mustard
⅓ c. prepared salsa

½ lb. lean (15% or less fat) ground beef
½ lb. lean ground turkey
1 c. soft bread crumbs
1 c. chunky salsa
¼ c. nonfat milk
2 eggs, beaten
½ tsp. salt
½ tsp. pepper

1 lb. lean flank steak, trimmed of fat
½ tsp. salt
1 tsp. cracked or freshly ground pepper
1 tsp. bottled minced garlic
1 tsp. olive oil
2 tsp. balsamic vinegar
1 ½ tbsp. fresh lemon juice

SALSA MEAT LOAF

Preheat oven to 400° F. In large bowl, combine all ingredients; mix well to form a loaf. Place loaf in foil-lined 5x9-inch baking pan; bake 40 to 45 minutes or until done. Serves 4.

Serve each with ¾ cup **Garlic Mashed Potatoes** and 1 cup **Sautéed Snap Peas.**
Exchanges: 3 meats, 2 breads, 2 vegetables, 2 fats

SALSA BEEF AND TURKEY LOAF

Preheat oven to 350° F. Combine all ingredients in large bowl; mix well. Form into a loaf and place on a rack placed over a pan (to allow fat to drain off). Bake 1 hour; let sit 10 minutes before slicing. Cut into 4-ounce slices; garnish with additional salsa. Serves 4. Refrigerate leftovers for sandwiches later in the week.

Serve each with ½ cup **Garlic Mashed Potatoes** and ½ cup cooked green beans.
Exchanges: 3 meats, 2 breads, 1 vegetable, 1 fat

FLANK STEAK

Rub steak with salt, pepper and garlic. Heat oil in large skillet over medium-high heat. Add steak; cook 6 minutes each side, or until desired doneness, basting with vinegar while cooking. Cut steak across grain into thin slices; drizzle lemon juice over pieces. Serves 4.

Serve each with 1 **Twice-Baked Potato** and 1 cup steamed broccoli.
Exchanges: 3 meats, 2 breads, 1 vegetable, 1 fat

GROUND BEEF STROGANOFF WITH NOODLES

Cook noodles according to package directions, omitting salt and fat. Drain and combine with ½ cup beef broth in medium cooking pot. Cook ground beef in skillet over medium heat until well done. Drain and remove from skillet; set aside. Using same skillet, sauté onion and mushrooms in margarine 3 minutes or until tender-crisp. Sprinkle with flour; season with salt and pepper. Add remaining beef broth; bring to a boil and simmer for 2 minutes. Add cooked ground beef and slowly stir in sour cream. Return to low heat and cook until warm—do not let boil or sour cream will curdle. Serve over noodles. Serves 4.

Serve each with 2 cups spinach salad tossed with 2 tablespoons low-fat sweet-and-sour dressing, and ¼ cup sliced strawberries.

Exchanges: 3 meats, 2 breads, 1 vegetable, ¼ fruit, 1 fat

1 lb. extra lean ground beef
6 oz. uncooked egg-free noodles
1 c. beef broth, divided
1 medium onion, diced
1 8-oz. pkg. sliced mushrooms
1 tbsp. reduced-fat margarine
1 tsp. flour
½ tsp. salt
½ tsp. black pepper
¾ c. reduced-fat sour cream

TEXAS ROUND STEAK

In shallow dish, blend flour, salt and 1½ teaspoons chili powder. Dredge meat in flour mixture (you'll use about half of the mixture). Place oil in heavy skillet; heat to frying temperature over moderate heat. Add meat; brown on both sides. Transfer steaks to 1½-quart casserole dish; set aside. Use skillet to sauté pepper and onion, stirring frequently; remove with slotted spoon and spread over meat. Drain remaining fat from skillet; add beef broth. Cook over moderate heat to loosen brown particles remaining in skillet. Add tomato juice, remaining 1 teaspoon chili powder, garlic powder and ground cumin; mix well and pour over meat. Use fork to lightly distribute broth and vegetables over meat. Cover tightly; bake at 325° F for 1 to 1½ hours or until meat is tender. Top each serving of steak with sauce. Serves 6.

Serve each with 1 cup **Roasted Potatoes** and 1 cup sautéed squash.

Exchanges: 3 meats, 2 breads, 2 vegetables, 1 fat

1½ lbs. beef round steak, cut into 6 pieces
½ c. all-purpose flour
1 tsp. salt
2½ tsp. chili powder
1 tbsp. vegetable oil
½ c. chopped green bell pepper
½ c. chopped onion
1 c. fat-free beef broth
½ c. tomato juice
¼ tsp. garlic powder
¼ tsp. ground cumin

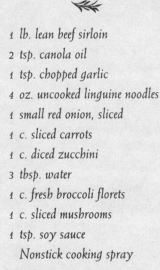

BEEF STIR-FRY

1 lb. lean beef sirloin

2 tsp. canola oil

1 tsp. chopped garlic

4 oz. uncooked linguine noodles

1 small red onion, sliced

1 c. sliced carrots

1 c. diced zucchini

3 tbsp. water

1 c. fresh broccoli florets

1 c. sliced mushrooms

1 tsp. soy sauce

Nonstick cooking spray

Heat oil over high heat in skillet sprayed with cooking spray. Add beef and garlic; stir-fry until cooked to your liking. Remove from skillet; keep warm. Cook noodles according to package directions, omitting salt and fat. Drain and keep warm. Stir-fry onion and carrots until carrots are partially done, adding water as needed to prevent sticking. Add zucchini, broccoli, mushrooms and soy sauce. (**Note:** Any combination of vegetables may be used.) Stir-fry until vegetables are done to your liking; add beef to reheat; then toss with pasta. Serves 4.

Serve with a 1-ounce breadstick and 1 cup sliced strawberries topped with 1 tablespoon nondairy whipped topping.
Exchanges: 3 meats, 2 breads, 1 vegetable, 1 fruit, 1 fat

BEEF STROGANOFF

1 lb. top sirloin, fat removed, cut in strips

2 tsp. canola oil

2 tbsp. chopped onion

$\frac{1}{4}$ c. sliced green onion tops

2 tbsp. all-purpose flour

1 c. beef bouillon

1 tsp. granulated garlic

$\frac{1}{8}$ tsp. black pepper

1 tbsp. tomato sauce

1 4-oz. can sliced mushrooms

$\frac{1}{2}$ c. reduced-fat sour cream

Nonstick cooking spray

Preheat medium skillet; coat with cooking spray. Brown meat and onion over medium heat. While meat is browning, combine flour and beef bouillon in covered container and shake well to remove all lumps; add to skillet along with garlic, pepper and tomato sauce. Cook over medium heat until sauce is thickened and meat is cooked to desired doneness, stirring constantly. Add drained mushrooms; stir in sour cream and blend until heated through—do not boil or sour cream will curdle. Serves 4.

Serve each with 1 cup cooked egg noodles, 4 tomato wedges topped with 1 teaspoon grated Parmesan cheese and 2 teaspoons **Balsamic Vinaigrette**, and 1 pear.
Exchanges: 3 meats, 2 breads, 1 vegetable, 1 fruit, 1 fat

GRILLED FILET MIGNON

3-oz. filet mignon per person, grilled to your liking.

Serve each with ½ cup steamed broccoli and a 6-ounce baked potato topped with 1 teaspoon reduced-fat margarine, 1 teaspoon salsa and 1 teaspoon reduced-fat sour cream.

Exchanges: 3 meats, 2 breads, 1 vegetable, 1 fat

BEEF KABOBS

Skewer meat and vegetables in following order: mushroom, meat cube, onion, zucchini, bell pepper, meat, onion, zucchini, bell pepper, meat, onion, zucchini, bell pepper, meat and mushroom. Place kabobs in 13x9-inch glass dish; set aside. In small bowl, combine oil, Worcestershire sauce, oregano and pepper; mix well and pour over kabobs. Cover dish and refrigerate overnight. Grill to desired doneness and garnish each with 3 cherry tomatoes. Serves 4.

Serve each with ½ cup grilled red potatoes, a 1-ounce slice of toasted French bread and ½ cup boiled baby carrots sprayed with butter-flavored cooking spray.

Exchanges: 3 meats, 2 breads, 2 vegetables, ½ fat

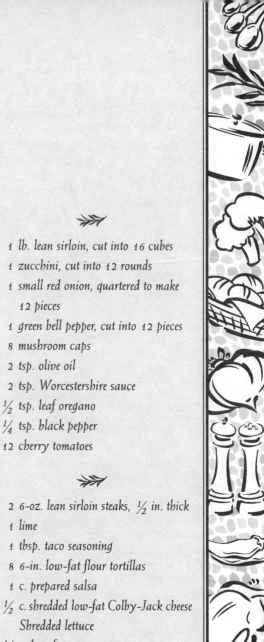

1 lb. lean sirloin, cut into 16 cubes
1 zucchini, cut into 12 rounds
1 small red onion, quartered to make 12 pieces
1 green bell pepper, cut into 12 pieces
8 mushroom caps
2 tsp. olive oil
2 tsp. Worcestershire sauce
½ tsp. leaf oregano
¼ tsp. black pepper
12 cherry tomatoes

STEAK TACOS

Preheat grill or broiler to medium-high. Squeeze lime juice over all surfaces of meat; then sprinkle each side with taco seasoning. Grill or broil to desired doneness (4 minutes each side for medium). While steaks are cooking, warm tortillas and salsa. Divide cheese evenly on top of steaks; cut each steak into 8 pieces. Serve 2 pieces of steak, garnished with shredded lettuce and sour cream. Serves 4.

Serve each with 2 low-fat tortillas, salsa, 1 cup **Marinated Cucumbers** and ¾ cup grilled fresh pineapple wedges (or canned spears).

Exchanges: 3 meats, 2½ breads, 1 vegetable, 1 fruit, 2 fats

2 6-oz. lean sirloin steaks, ½ in. thick
1 lime
1 tbsp. taco seasoning
8 6-in. low-fat flour tortillas
1 c. prepared salsa
½ c. shredded low-fat Colby-Jack cheese
Shredded lettuce
¼ c. low-fat sour cream

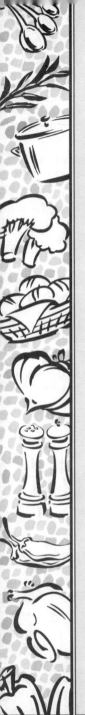

PASTA PRIMAVERA WITH MEAT SAUCE

1 lb. extra-lean ground beef

6 oz. uncooked penne pasta

¼ c. diced onion

¼ c. diced red or green bell pepper

1 c. sliced mushrooms

1 tsp. granulated garlic

1 tsp. salt

3 c. prepared spaghetti sauce

1 10-oz. pkg. frozen stir-fry
  vegetables, thawed

Nonstick cooking spray

Cook pasta according to package directions, omitting salt and fat. Drain and set aside. In large saucepan coated with cooking spray, sauté onion and bell pepper. Add mushrooms, garlic, salt and ground beef; cook 12 minutes or until done. Drain off excess fat; add spaghetti sauce and vegetables. Simmer for 5 minutes more; serve over pasta. Serves 4.

Serve each with 1 cup green salad tossed with 2 tablespoons low-fat dressing, and a 1-ounce breadstick.

Exchanges: 3 meats, 2 breads, 2 vegetables, ½ fat

GRECIAN SKILLET STEAKS

2 8-oz. lean strip-loin steaks, about
  1 in. thick

1½ tsp. crushed dried-leaf oregano

1 tsp. crushed dried-leaf basil

½ tsp. salt

¼ tsp. black pepper

1 tbsp. olive oil

3 garlic cloves, minced

2 tbsp. crumbled feta cheese

1 tbsp. fresh lemon juice

1 tbsp. chopped ripe olives

Sprinkle both sides of steaks with oregano, basil, salt and pepper. Heat oil to medium in large skillet. Add garlic; sauté 1 minute. Add steaks; cook 5 minutes each side for medium-rare (longer for well done). Remove from heat. Sprinkle with cheese, lemon juice and olives; cut each steak in half before serving. Serves 4.

Serve each with ½ cup **Roasted Potatoes**, 1 cup **Marinated Green Beans**, a 1-ounce dinner roll and 1 small orange.

Exchanges: 3 meats, 2 breads, 1 vegetable, 1 fruit, 1 fat

MEXICAN-STYLE BEEF AND PASTA

Cook pasta according to package directions, omitting salt and fat. Drain and set aside. Combine steak strips, taco seasoning, cilantro and garlic; toss to coat. Heat oil in skillet; sauté half of steak strips over high heat 1 to 2 minutes or until no longer pink. Remove with slotted spoon and repeat with remaining strips, removing all cooked strips from skillet. Add pasta, salsa, beans and water to skillet; cook 4 to 5 minutes over medium heat. Combine with steak in serving bowl; garnish as desired. Serves 4.

Serve each with ½ cup sliced cucumbers and ½ cup sliced bell peppers tossed with 2 tablespoons low-fat dressing, and 1 kiwi.
Exchanges: 3 meats, 2½ breads, 1½ vegetables, 1 fruit, 1 fat

1 lb. 1 in. thick round-tip steak, cut into ¼-in. thick strips

1 4-oz. pkg. uncooked rotini pasta

1 tbsp. olive oil

1 pkg. taco seasoning mix

1 tbsp. chopped fresh cilantro

3 garlic cloves, crushed

2 c. chunky salsa (any kind)

1 15-oz. can black beans, rinsed and drained

½ c. water

HEARTY VEGETABLE AND BEEF STEW

In medium saucepan, bring beef broth to boil. Cook 15 minutes or until reduced to 2 cups; remove from heat and set aside. In large Dutch oven, heat 1 teaspoon oil over medium-high heat. Add beef; brown on one side and remove from pan. Heat remaining oil in pan over medium-high heat; add onion, tomato paste and garlic; cook 5 minutes, stirring constantly. Return beef to pan; add reduced broth, carrots, potatoes, mushrooms, cooking wine, pepper and green beans. Bring to boil; cover, reduce heat and simmer 45 minutes or until vegetables are tender. In small bowl, combine water and cornstarch; stir well to remove lumps. Add to stew; bring to a boil and cook 1 minute, stirring constantly. Ladle 2 cups of stew into each soup bowl; garnish with parsley, if desired. Serves 4.

Serve each with 1 cup salad with 2 tablespoons low-fat dressing.
Exchanges: 2 meats, 2 breads, 2 vegetables, 1 fat

¾ lb. boneless, lean chuck roast, trimmed of fat and cut into ½-in. cubes

2 14¼-oz. cans fat-free beef broth

2 tsp. olive oil, divided

1 large onion, sliced

⅓ c. tomato paste

3 garlic cloves, minced

3 c. cubed carrots

3 c. cubed red potatoes

2½ c. quartered mushrooms

½ c. red cooking wine

¼ tsp. pepper

1 8-oz. can cut green beans

2 tbsp. water

1 tbsp. cornstarch

Chopped fresh parsley (optional)

½ lb. lean (15% or less fat) ground beef
½ c. chopped onion
1 ½ garlic cloves, crushed
4 oz. sliced mushrooms
½ c. spaghetti sauce
Dash pepper
½ 28-oz. can whole tomatoes,
   undrained and chopped
2 ½ tbsp. all-purpose flour
1 ¼ c. nonfat evaporated milk
½ c. crumbled feta cheese
½ c. shredded part-skim mozzarella
   cheese
2 c. uncooked penne pasta
1 ½ tsp. chopped fresh parsley (optional)

8 oz. cooked deli-style roast beef,
   thinly sliced
4 2-oz. hoagie-style rolls
1 teaspoon olive oil
1 ½ c. sliced onion
1 ½ c. sliced green bell pepper
¼ tsp. black pepper
4 1-oz. slices reduced-fat Swiss cheese
   Olive-oil-flavored nonstick
   cooking spray

CHEESE AND HAMBURGER CASSEROLE

THE DAY BEFORE, combine ground beef, onion and garlic in large nonstick skillet; cook over medium-high heat until browned, stirring to crumble meat. Add mushrooms; cook 5 minutes more or until tender. Add spaghetti sauce, pepper and tomatoes; stir well. Bring to a boil; reduce heat and simmer uncovered for 20 minutes. Set aside. Place flour in medium saucepan. Gradually add milk, stirring with a whisk until blended. Cook over medium heat 10 minutes or until thick, stirring constantly. Stir in cheeses; cook 3 minutes or until cheeses melt, stirring constantly. Reserve ½ cup cheese sauce; pour remainder along with beef mixture and pasta into 13x9-inch baking dish. Stir gently; drizzle reserved cheese sauce over top. Cover and refrigerate 24 hours.

NEXT DAY, preheat oven to 350° F. Bake, covered for 1 hour and 10 minutes or until thoroughly heated and pasta is tender. Garnish with parsley, if desired. Serves 4.

Serve each with a 1-ounce breadstick.
Exchanges: 2½ meats, 2 breads, 2 vegetables, ½ milk, 2 fats

PHILLY CHEESE BEEF SANDWICH

Preheat broiler. Heat oil in nonstick skillet over medium heat. Add onion; sauté 10 minutes, stirring frequently. Add bell pepper and black pepper; sauté 3 minutes more or until bell pepper is tender-crisp. Fill each roll with 2 ounces beef and ¼ cup sautéed vegetables topped with 1 slice cheese. Place sandwiches on baking sheet coated with cooking spray; broil 2 minutes or until cheese melts.

Serve each with 1 cup **Broccoli Slaw.**
Exchanges: 3 meats, 2 breads, 1½ vegetables, 1 fat

BBQ STEAK KABOBS

Preheat grill to medium. In large bowl, combine ketchup, molasses, Worcestershire sauce, mustard and onion; season with salt to taste. Add meat; toss to coat well. Thread steak chunks onto long skewers; grill to desired doneness (10 minutes for medium rare), turning occasionally and brushing with sauce. While skewers are cooking, toast French bread. Lightly rub one side of hot toasted bread with cut side of garlic clove. Serves 4.

Serve each with 1 cup grilled vegetables and ½ cup **Roasted Potatoes**.
Exchanges: 3 meats, 2 breads, 2 vegetables, 1 fat

1 ¼ lbs. boneless-round or top-sirloin steaks, trimmed of fat and cut into 2-in. pieces

2 tbsp. plus 2 tsp. ketchup

1 tbsp. light molasses

1 tbsp. plus 1 tsp. Worcestershire sauce

2 tsp. spicy brown mustard

2 tsp. grated onion

4 slices French bread, cut ½ in. thick, toasted and hot

1 garlic clove, halved

HEARTY BEEF STEW

Preheat oven to 450° F. Remove all visible fat from steak and cut into 1-inch pieces. In shallow dish, combine flour, salt and pepper; dredge steak in flour mixture and set aside. Coat a shallow baking sheet with cooking spray; transfer meat to pan and coat meat with cooking spray. Bake until meat is browned all over.

While meat is cooking, combine water, onion, bouillon, potatoes, celery, bay leaves, tomatoes, thyme, sage and carrots in a large saucepan; mix well and add meat. Bring mixture to boil; then cover and reduce heat. Simmer for 45 minutes, stirring occasionally. If mixture is not thick enough, thicken with a little cornstarch. Remove bay leaves before serving. Serves 4.

Serve each with 1 cup spinach salad with tomatoes and 2 tablespoons **Balsamic Vinaigrette**, and a 2x2-inch square of **Cornbread** or a 1-ounce dinner roll.
Exchanges: 2 meats, 2½ breads, 2 vegetables, 1½ fats

¾ lb. lean boneless top-round steak

2 ½ tbsp. all-purpose flour

⅛ tsp. salt

⅛ tsp. black pepper

2 c. water

¾ c. coarsely chopped onion

2 tsp. beef-flavored bouillon granules

¾ lb. new potatoes, quartered

3 stalks celery, cut diagonally into 1-in. pieces

2 bay leaves

1 28-oz. can stewed tomatoes

¼ tsp. dried leaf thyme

½ tsp. dried sage

2 large carrots, scraped and cut diagonally into 1-in. pieces

Nonstick cooking spray

ROSEMARY-SAGE STEAK

1 lb. boneless top sirloin steak,
  all visible fat removed
¼ c. fresh lemon juice
3 tbsp. dry white cooking wine
1 tbsp. Dijon mustard
1 tsp. olive oil
½ tsp. pepper
¼ tsp. salt
½ c. chopped onion
2 tbsp. finely chopped fresh rosemary
  (or 2 tsp. dried, crushed)
2 tbsp. finely chopped fresh sage
  (or 2 tsp. dried)
3 medium garlic cloves, minced
  (or 1 ½ tsp. bottled minced garlic)

Place steak in airtight plastic bag. In small bowl, combine all of remaining ingredients to create marinade. Pour marinade into bag with steak; turn to coat evenly. Seal bag and refrigerate at least 1 hour or up to 24 hours, turning occasionally.

Preheat grill to medium-high. Drain liquid from steak; grill 8 to 12 minutes per side or until desired doneness. Serves 4.

Serve each with 1 cup grilled vegetables and a 6-ounce baked potato topped with 1 teaspoon reduced-calorie margarine and 1 teaspoon reduced-fat sour cream.
Exchanges: 3 meats, 2 breads, 2 vegetables, 1 fat

GREEN PEPPER STEAK

1 lb. lean sirloin steak, cut into
  ¼-in. strips
2 tbsp. all-purpose flour
½ tsp. salt
¼ tsp. freshly ground pepper
1 tbsp. canola oil
1 15 ¾-oz. can beef broth
1 c. canned tomatoes, with juice
1 medium onion, sliced
1 garlic clove, finely chopped
1 large green bell pepper, cut into strips
1 ½ tsp. Worcestershire sauce

Mix flour with salt and pepper; coat strips of steak with flour mixture. Heat oil in large skillet. Brown meat on all sides; drain off any fat. Add broth, tomato juice (reserving the tomato pieces for later), onion and garlic. Cover and simmer 30 to 40 minutes or until meat is tender.

Add tomato pieces, green-pepper strips and Worcestershire sauce. Stir and cook 10 minutes longer. Serves 4.

Serve each over ½ cup cooked rice and with 1 cup cooked carrots.
Exchanges: 3 meats, 2 breads, 1 vegetable, 1 fat

DINNER MENUS WITH RECIPES

Beef

SEARED VEAL CHOPS WITH SUN-DRIED TOMATOES

Sear chops in large frying pan; add juice, water, Tabasco, salt and pepper. Cover tightly; simmer 15 minutes. Add sun-dried tomatoes; cook additional 10 minutes. Add 1 tablespoon basil. Cook 8 minutes; add remaining basil and cook 3 additional minutes. To serve, arrange the veal on a plate and spoon tomatoes and basil over top. Serves 4.

   Serve each with ½ cup **Fettuccine Alfredo**, ½ cup cooked mixed vegetables and a 1-ounce dinner roll.
Exchanges: 3 meats, 2 breads, 1 vegetable, 2 fats

4 lean, center-cut veal chops (1 ¼ to 1 ½ lbs.), excess fat removed
1 c. tomato juice
½ c. water
½ tsp. Tabasco sauce
   Salt and pepper to taste
¼ c. sun-dried tomatoes
2 tbsp. chopped fresh basil
   (or 1 tsp. dried)

PORK

CINNAMON-APPLE PORK TENDERLOIN

Preheat oven to 400° F. Place the tenderloin in roasting pan or casserole dish with a lid. In medium bowl, combine apples, cornstarch, cinnamon and raisins; stir. Spoon apple mixture around tenderloin. Cover and bake 40 minutes; remove lid and spoon mixture over top of tenderloin. Bake uncovered 15 to 20 minutes longer, or until tenderloin is browned and cooked through. Serves 4.

   Serve each with ½ cup brown rice and 1 cup cooked green beans.
Exchanges: 3 meats, 1 bread, 2 vegetables, 1 fruit

1 lb. pork tenderloin
2 apples, peeled, cored and sliced
2 tbsp. cornstarch
1 tsp. ground cinnamon
2 tbsp. raisins

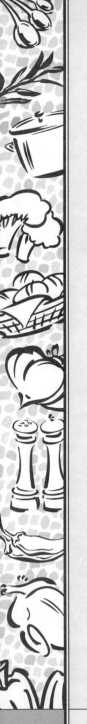

2 lbs. lean, boneless pork loin,
   cut into cubes
3 tbsp. flour
1 tsp. salt
1/4 tsp. dried thyme
1/4 tsp. pepper
3 c. sliced carrots
3 c. cubed potatoes
2 large onions, cubed
2 apples, cubed
2 c. apple cider
1 tbsp. vinegar
1/4 c. flour
1/2 c. cold water

4 4-oz. boneless pork loin chops
1/3 c. reduced-sugar orange marmalade
2 tbsp. Dijon mustard
1 bunch green onions, trimmed
2 c. mandarin oranges
   Nonstick cooking spray

CROCK-POT CIDER PORK STEW

In medium bowl, combine 3 tablespoons flour, salt, thyme and pepper; mix well. Add meat and toss to coat. Place carrots, potatoes, onion and apples in Crock-Pot; top with meat. In small bowl, combine apple cider and vinegar; pour over meat. Cover and cook 8 to 10 hours on low heat.

After stew is cooked, turn Crock-Pot setting to high. Combine 1/4 cup flour and cold water; blend well to remove lumps. Stir flour mixture into Crock-Pot; cover and cook 15 to 20 minutes or until thickened. Season to taste. Serves 8.

Serve each with 1 cup combined steamed broccoli and cauliflower and a 2-inch square of **Cornbread**.

Exchanges: 3 meats, 2 breads, 2 vegetables, 1 fat

ORANGE PORK CHOPS

Preheat broiler or outdoor grill to high. In a small saucepan, combine marmalade and mustard; heat to medium, stirring constantly until marmalade is melted; remove from heat and set aside. Drain juice from oranges; set fruit aside. Place chops on broiler pan. Broil about 4 inches from heat for 6 minutes; turn and broil 2 more minutes. Spoon half of marmalade glaze over chops; continue broiling 3 to 4 minutes more or until chops are no longer pink.

While meat is cooking, slice green onions diagonally into 1-inch pieces. Stir-fry in skillet coated with cooking spray 2 minutes or until tender-crisp. Stir in remaining glaze until heated and add oranges; serve over chops. Serves 4.

Serve each with 3/4 cup **Potato Salad** and 1 cup assorted grilled vegetables.
Exchanges: 3 meats, 2 breads, 1 vegetable, 1/2 fruit, 1 fat

PORK CHOPS WITH CHERRY SAUCE

Season pork chops evenly on both sides with garlic salt and pepper. Arrange in preheated skillet coated with cooking spray; brown well on both sides over medium heat. While chops are cooking, purée grape juice, vinegar, oregano, nutmeg and half the cherries in a blender. Pour purée over pork chops; sprinkle remaining cherries over top. Reduce heat; cover and simmer 10 minutes. Serves 4.

Serve each immediately with ⅓ cup cooked brown rice, 6 to 8 steamed asparagus spears and a 1-ounce slice of garlic bread topped with ½ teaspoon reduced-fat margarine.

Exchanges: 3 meats, 2 breads, 1 vegetable, 1 fruit, ½ fat

4 4-oz. boneless, center-cut pork chops, trimmed of fat
½ tsp. garlic salt
½ tsp. black pepper
½ c. red grape juice
½ tsp. balsamic vinegar
¾ tsp. crushed dried leaf oregano
½ tsp. ground nutmeg
1 16-oz. bag frozen, pitted dark red cherries, thawed and drained
Nonstick cooking spray

PORK TENDERLOIN AND VEGETABLE STIR-FRY

Preheat oven to 350° F. Place tenderloin in baking pan; drizzle soy sauce over top and bake for 1 hour. Let sit 10 minutes before slicing; then slice into approximately 1-ounce pieces. Divide quantity in half; set one half aside and then refrigerate other half to make BBQ-pork sandwiches another day. Heat oil in skillet; sauté vegetables until tender-crisp; add pork and heat through. Add teriyaki sauce and serve immediately. Serves 4.

Serve each with ⅔ cup cooked brown rice and 1 cup drained Dole tropical fruit (canned in light syrup).

Exchanges: 3 meats, 2 breads, 1 vegetable, 1 fruit, 1 fat

1 lb. pork tenderloin
2 tsp. soy sauce
2 tsp. canola oil
3 c. frozen stir-fry vegetables, thawed
2 tbsp. teriyaki sauce

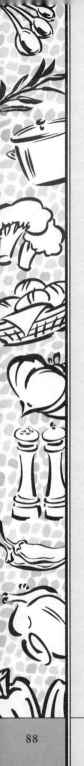

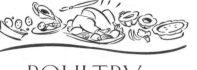

POULTRY

TURKEY STEAKS

4 3-oz. turkey mignon (cutlets)

1 tsp. canola oil

2 tsp. lemon-pepper seasoning, divided

½ c. reduced-fat ranch dressing

1 tbsp. prepared brown mustard

¼ tsp. dried dill

Heat oil in large skillet. Add cutlets; sauté over medium heat 8 to 10 minutes, turning occasionally. Add 1½ teaspoons lemon-pepper seasoning; sauté 2 minutes more, turning once. In small bowl, combine dressing, mustard, remaining lemon pepper and dill; mix well.

Serve each with ½ cup prepared herbed stuffing mix and 1 cup steamed cauliflower topped with 2 tablespoons sauce.

Exchanges: 2½ meats, 2 breads, 1 vegetable, ½ fat

MARMALADE CHICKEN

1 whole 3-lb. chicken, skin on,
   cut into 8 pieces

¼ c. orange marmalade

1 tbsp. soy sauce, diluted with
   1 tbsp. water

¼ c. fresh lemon juice

¼ tsp. crumbled dried thyme

¼ c. white cooking wine

Remove any visible fat from the chicken, but leave skin on. Combine marmalade, soy sauce, lemon juice, wine and thyme in medium bowl; mix well. Add chicken; turn to coat. Cover and marinate in refrigerator 4 hours, or overnight, turning occasionally.

Preheat oven to 400° F. Place a wire rack on top of a baking sheet. Remove chicken from marinade; set marinade aside. Place chicken, skin side up, on rack. Bake 50 minutes, turning every 20 minutes, resulting in final 10 minutes cooking skin side up, until skin is golden brown.

While chicken is cooking, boil marinade in small, heavy saucepan until reduced to glaze (about 10 minutes). Remove skin from cooked chicken and brush with glaze; bake until glaze is set and chicken is cooked through, approximately 5 minutes. Serves 4.

Serve each with 1 cup **Roasted Potatoes**, 1 cup **Sautéed Snap Peas** and a 1-ounce dinner roll.

Exchanges: 3 meats, 2 breads, 2 vegetables, ½ fat

CROCK-POT CHICKEN STEW

Combine all ingredients in Crock-Pot; cook on low heat 8 to 10 hours. Discard bay leaf before serving. Serves 4.

Serve each with a 2-inch square of **Cornbread**.
Exchanges: 3 meats, 2 breads, 2 vegetables, 1 fat

2 c. water

4 4-oz. boneless, skinless chicken breasts, cut into chunks

1 16-oz. can navy beans, drained

1 16-oz. can low-sodium stewed tomatoes

½ c. thinly sliced celery

1 ½ c. diced carrots

½ c. chopped onion

⅛ tsp. garlic powder

1 bay leaf

½ tsp. crushed dry leaf basil

¼ tsp. crushed dry leaf oregano

¼ tsp. paprika

1 tsp. low-sodium instant chicken or beef bouillon

GRILLED CHICKEN BREASTS WITH CORN SALSA

Combine sherry, soy sauce, cilantro, lime juice and jalapeños in medium bowl; mix well. Add chicken and turn to coat. Cover and marinate in refrigerator at least 1 hour, or up to 4 hours, turning occasionally.

Preheat barbecue or broiler to medium-high. Remove chicken from marinade; discard liquid. Season chicken with salt and pepper. Grill or broil chicken until cooked through, or about 4 minutes each side. Cut into thin diagonal slices; top each with **Corn Salsa**. Serves 4.

Serve each with 1 cup cooked green beans mixed with a little salsa, 2 cups spinach salad with mushrooms, tomatoes and 2 tablespoons low-fat dressing, and a 1-ounce dinner roll with 1 teaspoon reduced-calorie margarine.
Exchanges: 3 meats, 2 breads, 2 vegetables, ½ fat

4 4-oz. boneless, skinless chicken breasts

½ c. cooking sherry

1 tbsp. low-sodium soy sauce

1 tbsp. chopped fresh cilantro

2 tsp. fresh lime juice

1 to 2 tsp. seeded and chopped jalapeño peppers

Salt and pepper to taste

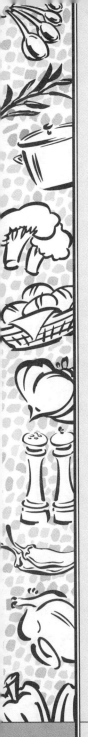

ORIENTAL CHICKEN AND CABBAGE SALAD

1 ½ lbs. cooked boneless, skinless chicken
    breasts, cubed

1 c. canned unsalted chicken broth

4 oz. snow peas, trimmed

⅓ c. rice-wine vinegar

4 large garlic cloves, minced

2 tsp. seeded and minced jalapeño
    peppers

1 tsp. oriental sesame oil

¼ c. chopped fresh cilantro

1 pkg. artificial sweetener

2 tbsp. soy sauce, diluted with 2 tbsp.
    water

3 tbsp. minced fresh ginger (or 1 tsp.
    ground)

5 ½ c. sliced Napa or green cabbage

4 ½ c. sliced red cabbage

2 c. sliced mushrooms

1 ½ c. grated carrots

1 c. chopped green onions

Bring broth to simmer in heavy, large skillet over medium heat. Add chicken and simmer until cooked through, or about 7 minutes. Remove chicken; set aside to cool. Add snow peas to broth and cook until tender or about 3 minutes. Using slotted spoon, transfer peas to bowl of cold water. Drain; set aside. Boil broth until reduced to ⅓ cup, or about 7 minutes. Remove from heat; set aside to cool.

Combine vinegar, garlic, jalapeño, sesame oil, cilantro, artificial sweetener, soy sauce and ginger in medium bowl. Add cooled broth and mix well. In large bowl, combine chicken, cabbage, mushrooms, carrots and onions; top with dressing mixture and toss well. Cover and refrigerate up to 6 hours. For a colorful presentation, arrange servings in red cabbage leaves. Serves 6.

Serve each with ¼ cup Chinese crispy noodles.
Exchanges: 3 meats, 2 breads, 2 vegetables, ½ fat

GRILLED SESAME CHICKEN

4 4-oz. boneless, skinless chicken breasts

2 tbsp. sesame seeds

3 garlic cloves, crushed

¼ tsp. freshly ground black pepper

1 tbsp. brown sugar

2 tbsp. soy sauce, diluted with
    1 ½ tbsp. water

Preheat grill to medium-high. Combine all ingredients except chicken in a shallow dish; mix well. Add chicken; turn to coat. Cover and marinate in refrigerator at least 2 hours. Drain chicken; grill 4 to 5 inches from coals for 15 minutes. Turn and grill until cooked through. Serves 4.

p140

Serve each with 1 cup **Sautéed Oriental Vegetables** and 1 cup cooked noodles tossed with 1 teaspoon teriyaki sauce.
Exchanges: 3 meats, 2 breads, 2 vegetables, 1 fat

SMOKED TURKEY QUESADILLAS

Place tortillas on flat work surface. Arrange cheese, turkey, grapes and cilantro over half of each tortilla. Sprinkle with cumin; fold tortilla over filling.

Preheat oven to 200° F. Heat large, nonstick skillet to medium. Spray hot skillet with cooking spray. Cook quesadillas one at a time for 3 minutes or until golden brown, turning once. Brush cooked top with lime juice and sprinkle with coarse salt. Cook until both sides are golden brown. Keep warm in oven while repeating process with remaining quesadillas. Serves 6.

Serve each with ½ cup chunky salsa mixed with 1 teaspoon reduced-fat sour cream.

Exchanges: 3 meats, 2 breads, 1 vegetable, ½ fruit, 1 fat

12 oz. 98% fat-free smoked turkey, sliced
6 7-in. low-fat flour tortillas
6 oz. low-fat Monterey-Jack cheese, grated
36 green grapes, halved lengthwise
   Fresh cilantro sprigs, stemmed
½ tsp. ground cumin
1 tbsp. fresh lime juice
½ tsp. coarse salt
   Nonstick cooking spray

SPICY WHITE-BEAN-AND-CHICKEN CHILI

(**Note:** May be made 3 days ahead. Cover and refrigerate. Reheat when ready to serve.)

Heat oil in large, heavy pot over medium heat. Add onion and garlic; sauté 10 minutes or until tender. Stir in cumin and oregano and cook 1 minute. Mix in beans, chilies, chicken, broth and water. Simmer until beans are very tender and chili is creamy (about 1 hour and 45 minutes or less).

Ladle chili into bowls; garnish with yogurt, cilantro and jalapeños, if desired. Serve immediately. Serves 4.

Serve each with 1 cup spinach salad with 2 tablespoons low-fat dressing.

Exchanges: 3 meats, 2 breads, 1 vegetable, ½ milk, 1 fat

¾ lb. boneless, skinless chicken breast, trimmed of fat and cut into large pieces
2 tsp. olive oil
1 extra-large onion, chopped
8 large garlic cloves, minced
1 tbsp. ground cumin
½ tsp. crumbled dried oregano
2 16-oz. cans navy beans
2 4-oz. cans diced green chilies
5 ¼ c. canned, unsalted chicken broth
¾ c. water
¾ c. plain nonfat yogurt
3 jalapeños, minced (optional)
   Chopped fresh cilantro, to taste

1 ½ c. chopped cooked chicken
1 8-oz. low-fat sour cream
1 8-oz. plain nonfat yogurt
1 10¾-oz. can Healthy Choice
  cream of chicken soup
1 4-oz. can diced green chilies
12 6-in. low-fat flour tortillas
1 c. shredded reduced-fat cheddar cheese
¼ c. sliced green onion
  Nonstick cooking spray

1 lb. boneless, skinless chicken breasts,
  cut into chunks
  Salt and freshly ground pepper to taste
1 tbsp. canola oil
1 small onion, diced
2 garlic cloves, minced
1 large tomato, seeded and chopped
1 bay leaf
¼ tsp. leaf marjoram
1 c. frozen whole-kernel corn, thawed
10 whole cherry tomatoes

LIGHT CHICKEN ENCHILADAS

Heat oven to 350° F. Spray 13x9-inch (3-quart) baking dish with cooking spray. In medium bowl, combine sour cream, yogurt, soup and chilies; mix well. Spoon approximately 3 tablespoons mixture down center of each tortilla. Reserve ¼ cup cheese; sprinkle chicken, onions and remaining cheese on each tortilla. Roll tortillas and place in baking dish, seam side down. Spoon remaining sour-cream mixture over tortillas; cover with foil and bake 25 to 30 minutes or until hot and bubbly. Remove foil; sprinkle with reserved cheese. Return to oven and bake, uncovered, 5 minutes more or until cheese is melted.

Place each serving of two enchiladas on bed of shredded lettuce and top with chopped tomatoes. Serves 6.

Serve each with ½ cup salsa.
Exchanges: 3 meats, 2 breads, 1 vegetable, ½ milk, 1 fat

✓ ARGENTINE CORN CHICKEN

Lightly season chicken with salt and pepper. Heat oil in large, nonstick skillet. Add chicken; cook until tender, turning occasionally to prevent burning. Remove from skillet and set aside; keep warm. Sauté onion and garlic in same skillet. Add chopped tomato, bay leaf and marjoram; simmer for 10 minutes. Add corn, cherry tomatoes and chicken; heat through, mixing well. Serves 4.

Serve each with ⅓ cup brown rice and 1 cup steamed vegetables.
Exchanges: 3 meats, 2 breads, 2 vegetables, 1 fat

CHICKEN BREASTS WITH RASPBERRY SAUCE

Heat oil in large nonstick skillet. Sauté onion 2 minutes (do not brown). Remove from heat; set aside. Season flesh side of breast with salt and pepper; add to pan and cook over medium heat only until each side is lightly browned. Add juice; continue cooking 12 minutes or until chicken is cooked through. Remove chicken from pan; add onions and cook until liquid has a syrupy consistency. Add raspberries; heat through. Remove skin from chicken before serving and top each breast with sauce. Serves 4.

Serve each with ⅔ cup **Rice Pilaf** and 1 cup steamed broccoli topped with 1 teaspoon melted reduced-fat margarine.
Exchanges: 3 meats, 2 breads, 2 vegetables, 1 fruit, 1 fat

4 4-oz. boneless chicken breast halves, skin on
2 tsp. olive oil
1 red onion, thinly sliced
½ tsp. salt
¼ tsp. freshly ground black pepper
1 c. raspberry-apple juice
2½ c. fresh raspberries (or 1 c. frozen)

MUSTARD CHICKEN

Preheat oven to 350° F. On a cutting board, cover each breast with plastic wrap and pound with a meat mallet until ½ inch thick. Heat oil in large nonstick skillet; add garlic and cook for 2 minutes over medium heat. Add chicken breasts; brown 3 minutes on each side. Transfer chicken (not liquid) to 1½-quart shallow casserole dish; set aside.

Add cider, water, mustard, dill, salt and pepper to skillet; stir to mix with chicken drippings. Bring to a boil and cook 1 minute; pour over chicken. Cover and bake 20 minutes. Add parsley and baste chicken with sauce; bake an additional 5 minutes. Serves 4.

Serve each with ½ cup **Garlic Mashed Potatoes**, 1 cup **Sautéed Squash with Peppers** and a 1-ounce breadstick.
Exchanges: 3 meats, 2 breads, 2 vegetables, 1 fat

4 4-oz. boneless, skinless chicken breasts
1 tbsp. olive oil
2 garlic cloves, minced
½ c. apple cider
¼ c. water
2 tbsp. Dijon mustard
½ tsp. dried dill
½ tsp. salt
¼ tsp. black pepper
⅓ c. chopped fresh parsley

4 4-oz. boneless, skinless chicken
breasts, each cut into 4 strips
2 tsp. brown sugar
2 tbsp. Dijon mustard
2 c. chunky salsa
Nonstick cooking spray

1½ to 2 lbs. split chicken breasts, bone in
2 tbsp. nonfat milk
2 tbsp. onion powder
½ tsp. crushed dried thyme
¼ tsp. garlic salt
⅛ tsp. ground white pepper
½ tsp. cayenne pepper
⅛ tsp. ground black pepper
Nonstick cooking spray

4 4-oz. boneless, skinless chicken
breasts (you can substitute fish fillets)
½ c. **All-Purpose Breading Mix**
Nonstick cooking spray

SALSA CHICKEN

Preheat oven to 350° F. In small bowl, combine brown sugar, mustard and salsa; blend well and set aside. Arrange chicken in 9x9-inch baking dish coated with cooking spray. Bake uncovered 10 minutes; then turn each strip. Pour sauce over chicken; bake additional 8 to 10 minutes or until chicken is cooked through. Serves 4.

Serve each with 2 low-fat tortillas, shredded lettuce, diced tomatoes, 1 tablespoon reduced-fat sour cream and ¼ cup reduced-fat refried beans baked with 1 teaspoon part-skim mozzarella cheese on top.
Exchanges: 3 meats, 2½ breads, 1 vegetable, 1 fat

BAKED CAJUN CHICKEN

Preheat oven to 375° F. Rinse chicken and pat dry with paper towels. Cut off skin and discard. Spray 13x9x2-inch baking dish with cooking spray. Arrange chicken in dish, meat side up; brush lightly with milk. In small bowl, mix onion powder, thyme, garlic salt and white, cayenne and black peppers. Sprinkle mixture over chicken; bake 45 minutes or until chicken is cooked through. Serves 4.

Serve each with ½ cup steamed rice and ½ cup steamed vegetables.
Exchanges: 3 meats, 1 bread, 1 vegetable, 1 fat

OVEN-FRIED CHICKEN (OR FISH)

Preheat oven to 425° F. Place breading in a shallow pan. Spray each breast (or fillet) with cooking spray and coat each side with breading mixture. Arrange in 9x9-inch baking dish coated with cooking spray. Bake 15 to 20 minutes. Serves 4.

Serve each with 1 cup steamed sugar snap peas and a 3-ounce baked potato topped with 1 teaspoon each reduced-fat margarine and reduced-fat sour cream.
Exchanges: 3 meats, 1½ breads, 1 vegetable, 1 fat

WHITE TURKEY CHILI

In 3-quart saucepan, sauté onion, bell pepper and garlic in oil over medium heat until tender. Add cumin, oregano, chili powder, cayenne pepper and salt. Cook for 1 minute. Stir in turkey, beans and broth. Bring to a boil; reduce heat and simmer uncovered for 30 minutes or until slightly thickened. Serves 4.

Serve each with 8 crackers and 1 cup green salad with 2 tablespoons low-fat dressing.
Exchanges: 3 meats, 2 breads, 1 vegetable, ½ fat

2 c. cooked light turkey meat, cubed
½ tsp. olive oil
1 ½ c. chopped onion
½ c. chopped green bell pepper
2 garlic cloves, minced
1 tsp. cumin
1 tsp. oregano
1 tsp. chili powder
¼ tsp. cayenne pepper
¼ tsp. salt
1 17-oz. can cannellini (white kidney beans), drained and rinsed
1 c. chicken broth

SPICY THAI CHICKEN

Preheat broiler. Use food processor to puree bell pepper and vinegar; pour purée into saucepan. Add red-pepper flakes. Bring to a boil; then reduce heat to simmer. Cook 3 minutes more; remove from heat and let stand until cool. After purée cools, stir in artificial sweetener or sugar; set aside. Broil chicken breasts 10 minutes or until browned; turn and broil 5 minutes more.

Prepare serving platter with bed of hot cooked white or brown rice (or couscous). Remove chicken from oven; place atop bed of rice. Spoon sauce over breasts; garnish with lime wedges and serve immediately. Serves 4.

Serve each with ⅔ cup rice and 1 cup **Sautéed Snap Peas**.
Exchanges: 2 meats, 2 breads, 1 vegetable, ½ fat

2 4-oz. boneless, skinless chicken breasts
1 small red bell pepper, chopped
2 tbsp. white vinegar
¼ tsp. crushed red-pepper flakes
1 pkg. Sweet & Low (or 2 tsp. sugar)
1 lime, sliced into 6 wedges

1 lb. boneless, skinless chicken breasts,
   cut into strips
1 tbsp. canola oil
1 medium onion, chopped
1 tbsp. chopped garlic
1 tbsp. curry
2 c. diced Granny Smith apples
¼ tsp. salt (optional)
½ c. raisins
1 ½ c. chicken broth, divided
2 tbsp. all-purpose flour
⅛ tsp. black pepper

1 lb. boneless, skinless chicken breasts,
   cut into 1-in. strips
2 tsp. canola oil
3 tbsp. lime juice
½ tsp. ground cumin
½ tsp. chili powder
1 green bell pepper, sliced
1 medium onion, sliced
8 6-in. low-fat flour tortillas
   Nonstick cooking spray

CHICKEN CURRY

Heat oil in skillet to medium; add chicken, onion and garlic. Stir-fry until chicken is browned. Add curry, apple, raisins, salt and 1 cup broth. Cover and simmer for 10 minutes or until chicken is done.

While chicken is cooking, combine flour and remaining broth in small bowl; whisk until smooth. Stir into chicken mixture and bring to a boil, stirring constantly until thickened. Serves 4.

Serve each over ½ cup cooked brown rice with 1 cup cooked green beans and 1 slice toasted diet whole-wheat bread cut into 4 triangles.
Exchanges: 3 meats, 2 breads, 1 vegetable, 1 fruit, 1 fat

CHICKEN FAJITA DINNER

In small bowl, mix oil, lime juice, cumin and chili powder; pour over chicken. Add vegetables; toss to coat. Heat skillet to medium-high. Coat with cooking spray; add chicken mixture and stir-fry until chicken is cooked through. In separate skillet, heat tortillas and fill each with chicken mixture. Serves 4.

Serve each with ½ cup salsa and 2 tablespoons reduced-fat sour cream.
Exchanges: 3 meats, 2 breads, 1 vegetable, 1 fat

YOGURT CUMIN CHICKEN

Preheat oven to 350° F. Arrange chicken in 9x9-inch pan coated with cooking spray. Bake uncovered for 20 minutes. In small bowl, mix yogurt, jam and cumin; spoon over chicken. Bake for additional 10 minutes. Garnish with grapes prior to serving. Serves 4.

Serve each with ¾ cup cooked pasta topped with ½ cup **Marinara Sauce**, **Baked Zucchini** and a 1-ounce dinner roll.

Exchanges: 3 meats, 2½ breads, 2 vegetables, 1 fruit, ½ milk, ½ fat

4 4-oz. boneless, skinless chicken breasts
8 oz. plain nonfat yogurt
3 tbsp. all-fruit apricot jam
1 tsp. ground cumin
1 c. seedless green grapes
Nonstick cooking spray

CHICKEN PITA SANDWICHES

THE DAY BEFORE, place chicken breasts, lemon juice, oil, garlic, curry and salt and pepper in large zip-top plastic bag; seal and shake well to coat chicken. Marinate in refrigerator overnight, turning bag occasionally.

NEXT DAY, combine cucumber, onion, mint and yogurt in a bowl; stir well. Cover and chill. Spray BBQ grill rack with cooking spray; preheat grill. Remove chicken from bag, reserving marinade. Grill chicken 10 minutes each side or until done, basting occasionally with reserved marinade. Let cool. Cut diagonally across grain into ¼-inch slices; set aside. Spoon 1 tablespoon lettuce, 1 tablespoon tomato and 1½ tablespoons yogurt sauce into each pita half; top with chicken. Serves 4.

Serve each with ½ cup carrot sticks and 2 tablespoons low-fat ranch dressing.

Exchanges: 3 meats, 2½ breads, 1 vegetable, 1 fat

1 lb. boneless, skinless chicken breasts
⅓ c. fresh lemon juice
¾ tsp. olive oil
1½ garlic cloves, minced
½ tsp. curry powder
Dash salt and pepper
1 c. thinly sliced cucumber
½ c. thinly sliced onion, separated into rings
1½ tsp. minced fresh mint
½ 8-oz. carton plain low-fat yogurt
4 6-in. whole-wheat pita bread rounds, cut in half
½ c. thinly sliced romaine lettuce
½ c. chopped tomato
Nonstick cooking spray

4 4-oz. boneless, skinless chicken breasts
½ c. chopped onion
½ c. chopped celery
1 ½ c. chicken broth
4 c. packaged seasoned stuffing mix
⅛ tsp. black pepper
1 10-oz. can reduced-fat mushroom soup
½ c. water
Nonstick cooking spray

4 3-oz. boneless, skinless chicken breasts
¼ tsp. granulated garlic
⅛ tsp. black pepper
1 c. prepared spaghetti sauce
¼ c. grated part-skim mozzarella cheese
¼ c. grated Parmesan cheese
Nonstick cooking spray

4 3-oz. boneless, skinless chicken breasts
4 thin slices low-fat ham (about ½ oz. each)
½ c. cornflake crumbs
½ tsp. paprika
⅛ tsp. black pepper
2 tbsp. nonfat milk
2 oz. Swiss cheese, sliced
Nonstick cooking spray

STUFFED CHICKEN BREASTS

Preheat oven to 350° F. In large saucepan, combine onion, celery and broth. Simmer until vegetables are soft. Add stuffing mix and pepper; mix well and set aside. Place each breast between plastic wrap; pound each to about ¼ inch thick. Divide stuffing mixture; wrap each breast around stuffing. Place stuffed breasts in 9x9-inch pan coated with cooking spray. In small bowl, combine mushroom soup and ½ cup water; mix well and pour over chicken. Bake covered 30 minutes or until chicken is no longer pink. Serves 4.

Serve each with 1 cup **Broccoli Slaw.**
Exchanges: 3 meats, 2 breads, 2 vegetables, 1 fat

BAKED CHICKEN PARMESAN

Preheat oven to 350° F. Place chicken in 9x9-inch pan coated with cooking spray. Season with garlic and pepper. Bake for 12 to 15 minutes; then turn and cover with spaghetti sauce. Sprinkle with mozzarella; return to oven and bake an additional 10 minutes or until chicken is done. Top with Parmesan. Serves 4.

Serve each with ½ cup cooked shell macaroni topped with ¼ cup **Marinara Sauce,** and 1 cup steamed squash.
Exchanges: 3 meats, 2 breads, 1 vegetable, ½ fat

CHICKEN CORDON BLEU

Preheat oven to 400° F. Cut a pocket into each breast; stuff each with one slice of ham. In shallow dish, combine cornflake crumbs, paprika and pepper. Roll breasts in milk; then crumb mixture. Arrange breasts in 9x9-inch pan coated with cooking spray; bake for 25 minutes. Remove from oven; top each breast with ½ ounce of cheese. Return to oven and bake 3 to 4 minutes more. Serves 4.

Serve each with ¾ cup **Garlic Mashed Potatoes** and ½ cup cooked green beans.
Exchanges: 3 meats, 2 breads, 1 vegetable, 1 fat

CHICKEN FLORENTINE

Preheat oven to 350° F. Melt margarine in large nonstick skillet over medium heat. Sauté chicken breasts 3 to 4 minutes each side or until browned well. In medium saucepan, combine soup, mozzarella, nutmeg and pepper; cook over medium heat until cheese is melted. Line bottom of 13x9-inch baking dish with spinach; top with chicken in a single layer. Pour cheese sauce evenly over chicken; sprinkle with Parmesan and bake 12 to 15 minutes. Serves 4.

Serve each with $\frac{1}{3}$ cup brown rice, 1 cup steamed cauliflower, a 1-ounce dinner roll and 1 banana.
Exchanges: 3 meats, 2 breads, 2 vegetables, 1 fruit, 1 fat

4 3-oz. boneless, skinless chicken breasts
2 tsp. reduced-fat margarine
1 10¾-oz. can condensed reduced-
   fat cream of chicken soup
¼ c. shredded part-skim mozzarella cheese
⅛ tsp. ground nutmeg
⅛ tsp. black pepper
2 10-oz. pkg. frozen chopped spinach,
   thawed
2 tbsp. freshly grated Parmesan cheese

CHICKEN CACCIATORE

Coat a large skillet with cooking spray. Add chicken, tomatoes, tomato sauce, onion and Italian seasoning. Cover and simmer 25 to 35 minutes, stirring occasionally. Add peas; cook 10 minutes more. Serves 4.

Serve each with $\frac{1}{2}$ cup boiled red potatoes and $\frac{1}{2}$ cup steamed baby carrots.
Exchanges: 3 meats, 2 breads, 2 vegetables, ½ fat

1 2½-lb. whole chicken, quartered,
   skin removed
1 16-oz. can Italian-style tomatoes
   with peppers
1 8-oz. can tomato sauce
1 onion, sliced
1 tsp. Italian herb seasoning
2 c. frozen peas
   Nonstick cooking spray

GRILLED HAWAIIAN CHICKEN

Place chicken in glass bowl; set aside. In separate bowl, combine cooking sherry, pineapple juice, brown sugar and soy sauce; mix well. Pour over chicken; marinate overnight or up to 48 hours. Grill over medium heat until cooked through; remove skin before serving. Grill fresh pineapple slices for garnish. Serves 4.

Serve each with $\frac{2}{3}$ cup **Rice Pilaf** and 1 cup **Sautéed Snap Peas**.
Exchanges: 3 meats, 2 breads, 2 vegetables, 1 fruit

4 4-oz. boneless chicken breasts, skin on
½ c. cooking sherry
½ c. pineapple juice
1 tsp. brown sugar
¼ c. soy sauce
8 fresh pineapple slices

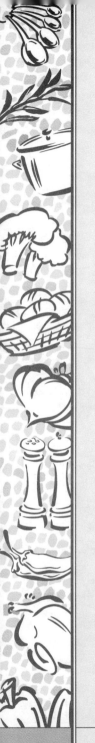

¾ lb. chicken tenders

2 10-oz. pkgs. frozen asparagus,
    thawed

1 10¾-oz. can reduced-fat cream
    of mushroom soup

½ c. low-fat mayonnaise

1 tbsp. lemon juice
    Dash cayenne pepper

¾ c. shredded reduced-fat
    cheddar cheese

¼ c. seasoned bread crumbs
    Butter-flavored nonstick
    cooking spray

12 oz. boneless, skinless chicken breasts,
    cut into bite-sized pieces

4 oz. uncooked linguine

½ c. chopped red bell peppers

½ c. chopped onion

½ c. sliced scallions

2 garlic cloves, minced

1 c. sliced mushrooms

1 tsp. crushed dry leaf oregano

2 c. broccoli florets

1 tbsp. reduced-fat margarine

½ c. evaporated nonfat milk

¼ c. shredded fresh Parmesan cheese

1 oz. reduced-fat Jarlsberg or Swiss
    cheese, shredded

ASPARAGUS CHICKEN

Preheat oven to 375° F. Coat 8x8-inch baking dish and large skillet each with cooking spray. Sauté half of chicken in skillet 1 to 2 minutes; remove and repeat with remaining chicken. Place asparagus in bottom of baking dish. Arrange chicken over asparagus. In medium bowl, combine soup, mayonnaise, lemon juice and pepper; mix well. Pour into skillet and heat until bubbly, stirring constantly. Pour over chicken; top with cheese, cover and bake 15 minutes. Remove cover and sprinkle with bread crumbs; bake uncovered 10 minutes more. Serves 4.

Serve each with ½ cup cooked rice and 1 small apple.
Exchanges: 3 meats, 2 breads, 1 vegetable, 1 fruit, ½ fat

CHICKEN LINGUINE

Cook linguine according to package directions, omitting salt and fat. Drain and set aside. Melt margarine in large nonstick skillet; sauté peppers, onions, garlic, mushrooms and oregano for 5 minutes or until tender-crisp. Add chicken, broccoli, margarine, milk and cheeses; cook until cheese melts, stirring constantly. Add linguine and mix well. Serves 4. (Refrigerate leftovers immediately for a great cold pasta salad.)

Serve with 1 cup **Fruit Salad** mixed with 1 tablespoon artificially sweetened vanilla-flavored nonfat yogurt.
Exchanges: 3 meats, 2 breads, 2 vegetables, 1 fruit, ¼ milk, ½ fat

CHICKEN RATATOUILLE

In large saucepan, sauté chicken in oil about 2 minutes per side. Add eggplant, zucchini, onion, mushrooms and bell pepper; simmer 10 minutes. Add tomato, thyme, basil, garlic and pepper; simmer 3 to 5 minutes. Serves 4.

Serve each with ⅔ cup cooked rice and 2 cups **Caesar Salad** with 2 tablespoons low-fat dressing.

Exchanges: 3 meats, 2 breads, 2 vegetables, 1 fat

4 4-oz. boneless, skinless chicken
  breasts, cubed
1 tbsp. olive oil
1 small eggplant, cubed
2 small zucchini, sliced
1 onion, sliced
½ lb. mushrooms, sliced
1 green bell pepper, sliced
1 large tomato, cubed
½ tsp. leaf thyme
1 tsp. leaf basil
½ tsp. granulated garlic
1 tsp. black pepper

SPICY CHICKEN STIR-FRY FETTUCCINE

Coat large nonstick skillet with cooking spray; set aside. In large pot, cook pasta according to package directions, omitting salt and fat. Drain well and leave in pot. In medium bowl, combine oil, garlic and pepper; mix well. Add chicken; toss to coat. Heat skillet over medium heat; stir-fry chicken 2 to 3 minutes. Remove from skillet with slotted spoon; sprinkle with salt and set aside. Add mushrooms to skillet; stir-fry 3 minutes. Add tomatoes and cooked chicken; stir well. Pour mixture into pot of pasta; heat if needed. Add cheese and toss well. Serves 4.

Serve each with 1 cup **Oven-Roasted Vegetables**.

Exchanges: 3 meats, 2 breads, 1½ vegetables, 1 fat

1 lb. chicken tenders
1 6-oz. pkg. uncooked fettuccine
2 tbsp. olive oil
3 garlic cloves, minced
¾ tsp. black pepper
½ tsp. salt
1 8-oz. pkg. sliced mushrooms
1 10-oz. can Rotel tomatoes
¼ c. freshly grated Parmesan cheese
  Nonstick cooking spray

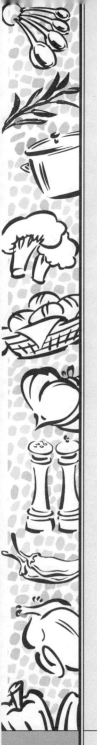

3 3-oz. boneless, skinless chicken
   breasts, cut into 16 strips
¾ c. shredded reduced-fat Swiss cheese
2 tsp. reduced-fat margarine
1 garlic clove, minced
1 c. sliced mushrooms
1 15-oz. can chunky tomato sauce
1 tsp. Italian seasoning
1 tbsp. all-purpose flour
2 tsp. sugar
   Butter-flavored nonstick
   cooking spray

4 3-oz. cooked boneless, skinless
   chicken breasts, cubed
2 tbsp. reduced-calorie margarine
½ c. all-purpose flour
¼ tsp. salt
¼ tsp. pepper
½ c. nonfat milk
1 10½-oz. can chicken broth
⅓ c. chopped onion
1 8½-oz. can cut green beans, drained
1 8¼-oz. can sliced carrots, drained
1 4½-oz. can refrigerated buttermilk
   biscuits

SWISS-STYLE CHICKEN

Preheat oven to 350° F. Place chicken in 8x8-inch baking dish coated with cooking spray; sprinkle cheese over chicken. Heat margarine in small skillet; sauté garlic 1 minute over medium heat. Add mushrooms; sauté 2 to 3 minutes or until tender. Combine tomato sauce, Italian seasoning, flour, sugar and mushrooms in small bowl; mix well and pour over cheese-topped chicken. Bake uncovered 30 to 35 minutes. Serves 4.

Serve each with ½ cup cooked rice and 1 cup steamed broccoli.
Exchanges: 3 meats, 1½ breads, 1½ vegetables, 1 fat

CHICKEN BISCUIT STEW

Preheat oven to 375° F. In heavy saucepan, melt margarine over medium-high heat; stir in flour, salt and pepper. Gradually add milk and broth, stirring with a whisk until blended. Cook 4 minutes or until thick and bubbly, stirring constantly. Add chicken, onion, green beans and carrots; cook 1 minute and remove from heat. Carefully split biscuits in half horizontally; place over chicken mixture to create topping. Bake 20 minutes or until biscuits are golden brown. Serves 4.
Exchanges: 2½ meats, 2 breads, 1 vegetable, 1½ fats

CALIFORNIA CHICKEN SALAD

Combine chicken, celery, carrots and almonds in medium bowl; set aside. In a small bowl, combine teriyaki baste and glaze, oil and vinegar mixture, sugar and ginger; pour about half of the dressing over the chicken mixture. Toss well to coat all ingredients. On four individual plates, evenly arrange cantaloupe wedges on top of the spinach; top each with chicken salad. Drizzle desired amount of remaining dressing over fruit and spinach. Serves 4.

Serve each with 6 slices melba toast.

Exchanges: **3 meats, 1 bread, 1 vegetable, ½ fruit, ½ fat**

1 ½ c. shredded cooked chicken breast

1 c. diced celery

1 c. julienned carrots

2 tbsp. slivered almonds, toasted

⅓ c. Kikkoman Teriyaki Baste and Glaze with Honey and Pineapple

1 tbsp. vegetable oil mixed with 1 tbsp. distilled white vinegar

1 tsp. sugar

1 tsp. minced fresh ginger root (or ¼ tsp. ground ginger)

1 medium cantaloupe, peeled and cut into 8 wedges

4 c. packed fresh spinach leaves

CHICKEN AND BROCCOLI FRITTATA

Preheat oven to 350° F. Cook broccoli in boiling water 3 minutes or until tender-crisp. Drain and set aside. Coat 9-inch pie pan with cooking spray; sprinkle with bread crumbs (do not remove excess crumbs); set aside. In large bowl, combine flour, basil, salt and pepper; add milk and mustard. Blend well with whisk; stir in egg substitute. Add chicken and ¼ cup cheese; stir well. Pour mixture into pie pan; sprinkle with remaining cheese and paprika. Bake 45 minutes or until set. Let cool on rack 5 minutes before slicing. Serves 4.

Serve each with 1 cup green salad with 2 tablespoons low-fat dressing, and 1-ounce dinner roll.

Exchanges: **3 meats, 1½ breads, 1 vegetable, 1 fat**

1 ½ c. chopped roasted chicken

2 c. chopped broccoli florets

2 tbsp. dry bread crumbs

3 tbsp. all-purpose flour

1 tsp. dried basil

¼ tsp. salt

⅛ tsp. pepper

1 c. nonfat milk

1 tsp. Dijon mustard

1 4-oz. carton egg substitute

½ c. shredded, reduced-fat, extra-sharp cheddar cheese, divided

¼ tsp. paprika

Nonstick cooking spray

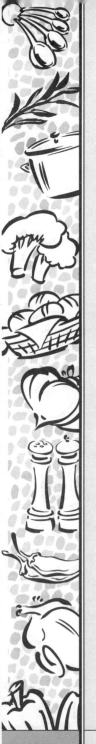

1 lb. boneless, skinless chicken breasts,
cut into 1-in. pieces
2 tsp. vegetable oil
1 ½ c. sliced mushrooms
½ c. chopped onion
1 garlic clove, minced
½ tsp. salt
½ tsp. dried basil
¼ tsp. pepper
2 c. coarsely chopped tomato
4 c. hot cooked fettuccine (about 8 oz.
uncooked)
¼ c. freshly grated Parmesan cheese

4 4-oz. boneless, skinless chicken
breasts
1 c. chicken broth
1 tbsp. water
½ tsp. cornstarch
½ 6-oz. tub reduced-fat cream cheese
with garlic and spices
3 c. hot cooked bowtie pasta
Chopped fresh parsley

CHICKEN AND FETTUCCINE

Heat oil in large nonstick skillet over medium-high heat. Add mushrooms, onion and garlic; sauté 2 minutes. Add chicken, salt, basil and pepper; sauté 5 minutes more or until chicken is cooked through. Add tomato; sauté 2 minutes more. Serve over pasta; sprinkle with cheese. Serves 4.

Serve each with 1 cup green salad with 2 tablespoons low-fat dressing.
Exchanges: 3 meats, 2½ breads, 1½ vegetables, 1 fat

CHICKEN AND BOWTIE PASTA

In large skillet, combine chicken and chicken broth. Bring to boil; cover, reduce heat and simmer 15 minutes, turning chicken after 8 minutes. Remove chicken from skillet; set aside and keep warm. Bring cooking liquid back to boil; cook 5 minutes or until reduced to ⅔ cup. In small bowl or cup, combine water and cornstarch; blend well and add to skillet. Bring to boil; cook 1 minute, stirring constantly. Add cream cheese; cook until well blended, stirring constantly with whisk. Serve each breast half over 3/4 cup pasta; then top with 3/4 cup sauce and garnish with parsley. Serves 4.

Serve each with 1 cup sautéed summer squash.
Exchanges: 3½ meats, 2½ breads, 2 vegetables, 1 fat

CHICKEN WITH GARLIC GRAVY

1 2-lb. whole chicken
1 tsp. dried thyme
¼ tsp. salt
¼ tsp. pepper
10 garlic cloves, peeled
½ c. white cooking wine
1 10½-oz. can low-salt chicken
   broth, divided
1 tbsp. all-purpose flour
   Nonstick cooking spray

Preheat oven to 325° F. Remove giblets and neck from chicken; discard. Rinse chicken under cold water; pat dry with paper towels. Trim excess fat. Starting at neck cavity, loosen skin from breast and drumsticks by inserting fingers, gently pushing between skin and meat. Rub thyme, salt and pepper on breasts and drumsticks under loosened skin; place 2 garlic cloves in body cavity. Lift wing tips up and over back; tuck under chicken. Set aside. Combine remaining garlic cloves, cooking wine and half of broth in shallow roasting pan lined with foil. Place chicken on cooking rack coated with cooking spray; place rack in foil-lined pan. Insert meat thermometer into meaty part of thigh, making sure not to touch bone. Bake 1 hour and 45 minutes or until thermometer registers 180° F. Discard skin; place chicken on a platter and set aside, reserving pan drippings. Keep chicken warm.

Place flour in small saucepan; gradually add remaining half of broth, stirring with whisk until blended; set aside. Place a small zip-top plastic bag inside 2-cup measuring cup. Pour pan drippings into bag; let stand 10 minutes (fat will rise to the top). Seal bag; carefully snip off bottom corner of bag. Drain drippings into broth mixture in saucepan, stopping before fat layer reaches opening; discard fat. Bring mixture to a boil; cook 1 minute or until thick, stirring constantly with a whisk. Arrange 3 ounces chicken topped with 3 tablespoons gravy for each serving. Serves 4.

Serve each with ⅔ cup mashed potatoes, 1 cup cooked green beans and a 1-ounce dinner roll.
Exchanges: 3 meats, 2 breads, 2 vegetables, ½ fat

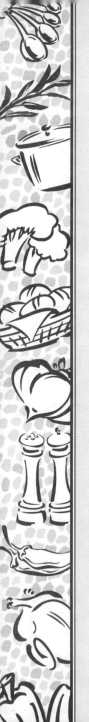

4 4-oz. boneless, skinless chicken
   breasts

2 tsp. vegetable oil

⅔ c. low-salt chicken broth

¼ tsp. salt

⅛ tsp. crushed red pepper

1 14½-oz. can Cajun-style stewed
   tomatoes, undrained and chopped

2 garlic cloves, crushed

1 10-oz. pkg. frozen cut okra, thawed

1½ tbsp. all-purpose flour

2 tbsp. water

¼ tsp. hot sauce (e.g., Tabasco)

2 c. hot cooked long-grain rice

¾ lb. ground chicken breast

1 15-oz. can Italian-style diced
   tomatoes, drained (reserve 3½ tbsp.
   juice)

¾ small onion, chopped

¾ small green bell pepper, chopped

1 clove garlic, minced

⅓ c. plain bread crumbs

1 egg

1¼ tsp. Italian herb seasoning

⅓ c. shredded fat-free mozzarella cheese

2 tbsp. freshly grated Parmesan cheese

CREOLE CHICKEN AND RICE

Heat oil in large nonstick skillet over medium-high heat. Add chicken; cook 2 minutes each side. Add broth, salt, pepper, tomatoes and garlic; cover, reduce heat and simmer 8 minutes or until chicken is done. Add okra; simmer, covered, 3 minutes more. In small bowl, combine flour and water, stirring with a whisk; add to skillet. Simmer, uncovered, 2 minutes or until thick. Stir in hot sauce. Serves 4.

Serve each with ¾ cup sauce and ½ cup rice.

Exchanges: 3 meats, 2 breads, 2 vegetables, ½ fat

CHICKEN CACCIATORE PIE

Preheat oven to 350° F. In medium bowl, combine reserved tomato juice, onion, bell pepper, garlic, bread crumbs and egg. Add half the Italian seasoning; salt and pepper to taste. Mix thoroughly. Add ground chicken; mix well. Pat mixture evenly into lightly oiled 10-inch pie plate, pushing up sides to form a shell. Bake 25 minutes.

In stainless-steel saucepan, combine tomatoes and remaining Italian seasoning; salt and pepper to taste. Simmer 10 to 15 minutes over medium heat; remove from heat and set aside. Remove meat shell from oven; discard excess liquid. Sprinkle shell with mozzarella. Add tomato sauce, sprinkle with Parmesan and bake 15 minutes until meat shell is cooked throughout. Let stand 5 minutes before cutting and serving. Serves 4.

Serve each with 1 cup green salad with 2 tablespoons low-fat dressing, and a 1-ounce slice toasted French bread.

Exchanges: 3 meats, 2 breads, 2 vegetables, 2 fats

CHICKEN AND PASTA PRIMAVERA

Place flour in shallow dish. Dredge chicken in flour; sprinkle with salt and pepper. Heat oil in large nonstick skillet coated with cooking spray. Add chicken; stir-fry over medium heat 4 minutes or until browned. Add mushrooms, broccoli, squash, carrots and garlic; stir-fry 2 minutes more. Stir in basil and tomatoes; spoon mixture into a large bowl; set aside. Add broth and wine to skillet, scraping pan to loosen browned bits; bring to a boil. Combine broth, chicken and pasta; toss well and sprinkle with cheese. Serves 4.

Serve each with 1 cup green salad with 2 tablespoons low-fat dressing.
Exchanges: 3 meats, 2½ breads, 2 vegetables, 1 fat

1 lb. boneless, skinless chicken breast, cut into bite-size pieces
⅔ c. all-purpose flour
¼ tsp. salt
¼ tsp. pepper
1½ tbsp. olive oil
1 c. sliced mushrooms
2 c. broccoli florets
2 c. sliced yellow squash
⅔ c. diagonally-sliced carrots
4 garlic cloves, minced
¼ c. chopped fresh basil
16 cherry tomatoes, halved
1 c. no-salt chicken broth
⅔ c. dry white wine
3 c. hot cooked linguine (about 3 oz. uncooked)
½ c. freshly grated Parmesan cheese
Nonstick cooking spray

BBQ CHICKEN BREASTS WITH APRICOT GLAZE

Preheat grill to medium. Grill chicken (skin on) 10 minutes, turning occasionally. Remove from grill and remove skin. In small bowl, combine preserves, soy sauce, water, ketchup and brown sugar; blend well. Return chicken to grill; generously brush with glaze. Continue cooking 10 to 15 minutes or until thoroughly done, turning often and brushing with glaze frequently. Serves 4.

Serve each with 1 cup mashed potatoes and 1 cup seasoned green beans.
Exchanges: 3 meats, 2 breads, 2 vegetables, 1 fat

4 chicken breasts (about 1½ lbs.), skin on and bone in
⅓ c. apricot preserves
1 tbsp. soy sauce
1 tbsp. water
2 tbsp. plus 2 tsp. ketchup
2 tsp. brown sugar

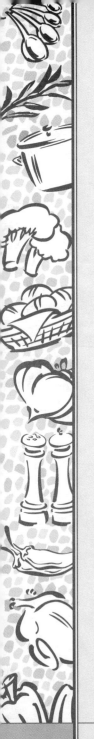

4 4-oz. boneless, skinless chicken breasts

3 garlic cloves, minced

1 small onion, thinly sliced

½ tsp. ground cumin

½ c. orange juice

1 tbsp. lemon juice

1 tsp. grated orange peel (orange part only)

¼ tsp. ground pepper

2 tsp. capers

Olive oil nonstick cooking spray

4 4-oz. boneless, skinless chicken breasts, cut crosswise into ¼-in. strips

½ lb. fresh asparagus spears, trimmed and cut into 1-in. lengths

2 medium carrots, cut into ⅛ in. thick rounds

1 small onion, thinly sliced

2 tbsp. reduced-fat margarine

2 tsp. lemon juice

½ tsp. tarragon

⅛ tsp. cayenne pepper

Salt and pepper to taste

CITRUS-BRAISED CHICKEN BREASTS WITH CAPERS

Rinse chicken and pat dry. Preheat nonstick skillet sprayed with cooking spray. Brown chicken on both sides over medium-high heat; remove from pan. Reduce heat and recoat pan with cooking spray. Add garlic; stir until browned slightly. Add onion; continue cooking, stirring until onion begins to brown. Stir in cumin, citrus juices, orange peel and pepper. Add chicken; cover and simmer for 10 minutes. Add capers and simmer covered, 5 to 8 minutes or until chicken is tender.

Top each breast with onions, capers and 1 tablespoon citrus sauce prior to serving. Serves 4.

Serve each with ⅔ cup cooked rice and 1 cup **Sautéed Snap Peas**.
Exchanges: 3 meats, 2 breads, 1 vegetable, ½ fat

CHICKEN BREASTS WITH ASPARAGUS AND CARROTS

Preheat oven to 450° F. Tear off 4 large pieces of aluminum foil (one for each serving). Arrange chicken in center of lower half of each length of foil. Season with salt and pepper; top with equal amounts of asparagus, carrots and onion. In small microwave-safe bowl, melt margarine; then add lemon juice, tarragon and cayenne pepper; salt to taste. Pour equal amounts of liquid over each serving of chicken. For each serving, fold two ends of foil together and tightly fold three or four times. Repeat process with ends to seal packet tightly. Arrange foil packets in a single layer on baking sheet; bake 20 minutes and serve. Serves 4.

Serve each with ½ cup cooked rice and a 1-ounce dinner roll.
Exchanges: 3 meats, 2 breads, 1 vegetable, 1 fat

CHICKEN AND GREEN BEAN DINNER

Preheat oven to 350° F. Place flour in oven-roasting bag. Add soup, green beans and chicken broth to flour; salt and pepper to taste. Squeeze bag to blend mixture. Place bag in baking pan and arrange ingredients in an even layer in bag. Sprinkle chicken with paprika; add salt and pepper. Place chicken and potatoes inside roasting bag on top of green bean mixture. Close bag and cut 4½-inch slits in top. Bake 45 to 50 minutes or until chicken is tender. Serves 4.

Serve each with 1 cup **Broccoli Slaw** and a 1-ounce dinner roll.
Exchanges: 3 meats, 2 breads, 2 vegetables, 1½ fats

2½ lbs. skinless chicken pieces, bone in
1 tbsp. all-purpose flour
1 11-oz. can reduced-fat cream of mushroom soup
1 10-oz. pkg. frozen green beans, thawed
½ c. chicken broth
⅛ tsp. paprika
¾ lb. potatoes, scrubbed and cut into 2-in. pieces
Salt and pepper to taste

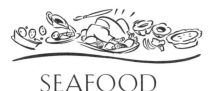

SEAFOOD

SHRIMP SCAMPI

Melt margarine and combine with oil, garlic, cooking wine and pepper in large bowl; mix well. Add shrimp and toss lightly to coat. In shallow casserole dish, spread shrimp in a single layer. (**Note:** The casserole dish must be oven safe, as it will be going in the broiler.) Broil shrimp approximately 4 inches from heat source 3 to 4 minutes. Turn and broil additional 3 to 4 minutes or until lightly browned. Sprinkle with parsley and serve. Serves 4.

Serve each with ½ cup **Fettuccine Alfredo** and 1 cup **Sautéed Snap Peas**.
Exchanges: 2 meats, 2 breads, 1 vegetable, 1 fat

1 lb. uncooked large fresh shrimp, deveined
1 tsp. margarine
1 tsp. olive oil
1 garlic clove, minced
¼ c. white cooking wine
¼ tsp. freshly ground black pepper
1 tbsp. chopped fresh parsley

3 low-fat Italian turkey sausages
(about 3 oz.), casings removed

¼ lb. small shrimp, deveined

2 4-oz. catfish fillets, each cut into
4 pieces

¼ c. all-purpose flour

1 tbsp. vegetable oil

1 c. chopped onion

1 c. chopped green bell pepper

3 garlic cloves, chopped

1 tsp. dried thyme

1 bay leaf

1 28-oz. can diced tomatoes

1 c. canned low-salt chicken or
vegetable broth

2 tsp. Creole or Cajun seasoning

1 ½ lbs. snapper fillets, cut into 4 6-oz.
portions

¼ c. lime juice

½ c. egg substitute

1 c. finely crushed ranch-flavored
tortilla chips

1 c. chunky salsa

¼ c. chopped fresh cilantro
Nonstick cooking spray

SEAFOOD AND TURKEY SAUSAGE GUMBO

Sprinkle flour over bottom of large, heavy pot. Stir constantly over medium-low heat until flour turns golden brown (do not allow to burn), or approximately 12 to 15 minutes. Pour browned flour into bowl; set aside.

Heat oil (using same pot) over medium heat. Add onion and bell pepper; sauté 7 minutes or until tender. Add garlic, thyme and bay leaf; cook 1 minute, stirring constantly. Add sausages; sauté about 5 minutes or until brown, breaking up with back of spoon. Add browned flour, tomatoes (with juice), broth and Creole/Cajun seasoning. Bring to boil. Reduce heat, cover and simmer 20 minutes to blend flavors, stirring frequently. Add shrimp and catfish; simmer 5 minutes or just until seafood is opaque in center. Discard bay leaf; season with salt and pepper and place each serving over ½ cup steamed rice. Serves 4.

Serve each with 1 cup green salad with 2 tablespoons low-fat dressing, and 4 saltine crackers.

Exchanges: 3 meats, 2 breads, 2 vegetables, 2 fats

SOUTHWESTERN SNAPPER

Preheat oven to 450° F. Rinse fillets with cold water and pat dry with paper towels. Combine lime juice and egg substitute in shallow dish. Place tortilla crumbs in separate dish. Dip each fillet into egg mixture; press into seasoned crumbs to coat. Place on baking sheet coated with cooking spray and sprinkle with any remaining crumbs. Bake 10 to 12 minutes or until fish flakes with fork. Top each fillet with ¼ cup salsa and garnish with cilantro. Serves 4.

Serve each with Broccoli Slaw and ½ cup Garlic Mashed Potatoes.
Exchanges: 3 meats, 2 breads, 1 vegetable, 1 fat

CITRUS SHRIMP SALAD

Bring water and seasoned salt to a boil; add shrimp. Cook 3 to 5 minutes; drain and rinse with cold water. Peel and devein shrimp; chill. In large bowl, combine dressing, shallots, vinegar, yogurt, orange juice, mustard, honey and pepper; mix well. Add shrimp and stir to coat. Line large platter with lettuce; spoon shrimp mixture into center of platter; arrange grapefruit sections and orange sections around salad. Garnish with chives. Serves 4.

Serve with 5 slices melba toast.

Exchanges: **2 meats, 1 bread, ½ vegetable, ½ fruit**

1 lb. medium shrimp, uncooked
   and unpeeled
1 qt. water
1 tbsp. seasoned salt
2 tbsp. low-fat Italian dressing
1 ½ tbsp. finely chopped shallots
1 tbsp. red wine vinegar
1 tbsp. plain nonfat yogurt
1 tbsp. orange juice
2 ¼ tsp. Dijon mustard
1 ½ tsp. honey
   Dash pepper
2 c. sliced romaine lettuce
1 c. pink grapefruit sections (about
   4 large grapefruit)
1 c. orange sections (about 5 oranges)
2 tbsp. chopped fresh chives

INDONESIAN SNAPPER FILLETS

Coat broiler rack with cooking spray; preheat broiler. Combine lemon juice, curry, sesame oil and yogurt in large zip-top plastic bag. Add fillets; seal and marinate in refrigerator 20 minutes. Remove fillets from bag and discard marinade. Arrange fillets on broiler rack; sprinkle with salt and pepper. Broil 8 minutes or until fillets flake easily with fork. Serves 4.

Serve each with 1 cup cooked linguine tossed with 2 teaspoons teriyaki sauce, and ½ cup **Sautéed Snap Peas**.

Exchanges: **3 meats, 2 breads, 1 vegetable, ¼ milk, 1 ½ fats**

4 4-oz. snapper fillets, about
   1 in. thick
¼ c. fresh lemon juice
1 tbsp. curry powder
1 tbsp. sesame oil
1 8-oz. carton plain nonfat yogurt
¼ tsp. salt
⅛ tsp. pepper
   Nonstick cooking spray

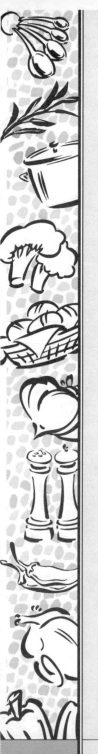

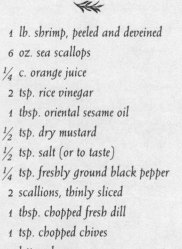

1 lb. shrimp, peeled and deveined

6 oz. sea scallops

¼ c. orange juice

2 tsp. rice vinegar

1 tbsp. oriental sesame oil

½ tsp. dry mustard

½ tsp. salt (or to taste)

¼ tsp. freshly ground black pepper

2 scallions, thinly sliced

1 tbsp. chopped fresh dill

1 tsp. chopped chives

4 lettuce leaves

1 ½ lbs. cod, tilapia, catfish or haddock
   fillets

¼ c. low-fat mayonnaise

1 tsp. Dijon mustard

1 tsp. white wine Worcestershire sauce

2 tsp. dried onion flakes

1 tsp. Old Bay seasoning

½ tsp. lemon-pepper seasoning

¼ tsp. paprika

⅛ tsp. cayenne pepper

1 tbsp. dried parsley (or 2 tbsp.
   chopped fresh)
   Nonstick cooking spray

STEAMED SHRIMP AND SCALLOPS

Arrange shrimp and scallops on a plate in a steamer basket. Sprinkle with 1 teaspoon orange juice and 1 teaspoon rice vinegar. Place steamer over boiling water in wok or large skillet and cover. Cook 7 to 8 minutes or until shrimp and scallops are cooked through.

While seafood is cooking, combine sesame oil, mustard, salt, pepper and remaining juice and vinegar in medium bowl; mix well. Add scallions, dill and chives. Transfer hot seafood to bowl with vinaigrette; toss to coat well. Serve warm on lettuce-lined plates; garnish with chopped pimiento if desired. Serves 4.

Serve each with 1 cup Roasted Potatoes, 1 steamed 6-inch ear corn on the cob and 1 cup cooked green beans.

Exchanges: 3 meats, 2 breads, 2 vegetables, 1 fat

QUICK BAKED FISH

Preheat oven to 400° F. Rinse fillets with cold water and pat dry with paper towels; place in shallow casserole dish sprayed with cooking spray. In small bowl, combine remaining ingredients until well mixed. Spread mixture evenly over fillets. Bake uncovered for 15 minutes or until fish flakes easily with a fork. Serves 4.

Serve each with ½ cup cooked brown rice, 1 cup steamed broccoli and a 1-ounce breadstick.

Exchanges: 3 meats, 2 breads, 1 vegetable, 1 fat

SALMON CAKES

Remove skin from fish. Combine all ingredients in a medium bowl, mashing salmon bones with fork. Shape into 4 cakes. Heat skillet to medium hot; spray with cooking spray. Cook salmon cakes until lightly browned, turning once. Serves 4.

Serve each with 1 cup **Summer Coleslaw** and a 1-ounce breadstick.
Exchanges: 2½ meats, 2 breads, 1 fat

1 15 ½-oz. can (2 c. flaked) red salmon, drained
1 tsp. onion powder
¼ c. diced red pepper or canned pimiento
4 drops Tabasco sauce
6 unsalted saltine crackers, crushed
3 tbsp. low-fat dressing or mayonnaise
   Nonstick cooking spray

SCALLOPS PARMESAN

Melt margarine in skillet over medium-high heat. Sauté garlic and scallops for 3 to 4 minutes; add lemon juice and stir. Set aside and keep warm. Use separate skillet to cook tomatoes 5 to 10 minutes or until slightly reduced. Add scallops to tomatoes; heat throughout. Top with cheese. Serves 4.

Serve each with ½ cup brown rice, 1 cup steamed broccoli and a 1-ounce dinner roll.
Exchanges: 3 meats, 2 breads, 1½ vegetables, 1 fat

1 ¼ lb. bay scallops
2 tbsp. reduced-fat margarine
1 garlic clove, chopped
2 tbsp. lemon juice
1 28-oz. can diced Italian-style tomatoes with juice
¼ c. shredded Parmesan cheese

LEMON FISH

Preheat oven to 450° F. Arrange fillets in 9x13-inch baking dish; top with remaining ingredients in order. Bake uncovered for 10 minutes per inch of thickness or until fish flakes easily. Serves 4.

Serve each with ¾ cup boiled red potatoes, spinach salad with 2 tablespoons low-fat dressing, ½ cup steamed asparagus with 1 teaspoon melted margarine, and a 1-ounce dinner roll.
Exchanges: 3 meats, 2 breads, 1 vegetable, 1 fat

1 lb. fish fillets (snapper, tilapia or catfish)
2 tsp. reduced-fat margarine
¼ c. chicken broth
⅛ tsp. black pepper
4 lemon slices
⅛ tsp. paprika
2 tsp. lemon juice
⅛ tsp. dried dill

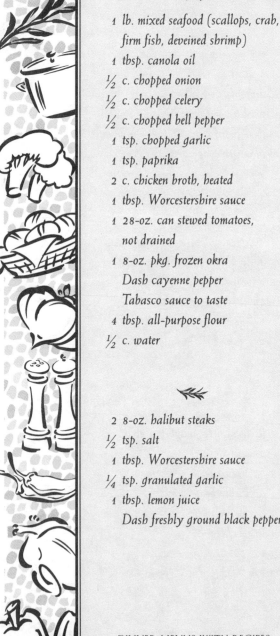

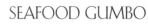

SEAFOOD GUMBO

1 lb. mixed seafood (scallops, crab, firm fish, deveined shrimp)
1 tbsp. canola oil
½ c. chopped onion
½ c. chopped celery
½ c. chopped bell pepper
1 tsp. chopped garlic
1 tsp. paprika
2 c. chicken broth, heated
1 tbsp. Worcestershire sauce
1 28-oz. can stewed tomatoes, not drained
1 8-oz. pkg. frozen okra
Dash cayenne pepper
Tabasco sauce to taste
4 tbsp. all-purpose flour
½ c. water

Use oil to sauté onion, celery and bell pepper in saucepan over medium heat. Cook until tender. Add garlic and paprika; sauté 1 minute more. Add 1 teaspoon flour; sauté 2 more minutes (do not let burn). Add heated broth and Worcestershire sauce; bring to a boil. Reduce heat; add tomatoes and okra. Let simmer over medium heat until vegetables are tender. Add cayenne pepper and Tabasco. Combine flour and water in a covered container; shake well to blend. Add to gumbo mixture and cook until bubbly and mixture thickens. Add seafood and continue to cook until seafood is cooked through. Serves 4.

Serve each over ½ cup cooked rice and 1 slice toasted French bread.
Exchanges: 3 meats, 2 breads, 2 vegetables, 1 fat

GRILLED HALIBUT STEAKS

2 8-oz. halibut steaks
½ tsp. salt
1 tbsp. Worcestershire sauce
¼ tsp. granulated garlic
1 tbsp. lemon juice
Dash freshly ground black pepper

In small bowl, combine all ingredients except for fish; set aside. Place fish in shallow dish and pour half of marinade over fish; turn to coat. Let marinate in refrigerator 1 hour; then grill or broil to desired doneness, basting with remaining marinade while cooking. Cut steaks in half. Serves 4.

Serve each with 1 cup steamed broccoli, ½ cup brown rice and a 1-ounce dinner roll with 1 teaspoon reduced-fat margarine.
Exchanges: 3 meats, 2 breads, 2 vegetables, ½ fat

SEAFOOD CREOLE

Heat oil and ½ cup chicken broth in saucepan using medium heat. Add onions; cook for 3 minutes. Add pepper and celery; cook an additional 3 minutes. Add spices, brown sugar, salt and garlic; let simmer 5 minutes. Whisk in flour; cook additional 3 minutes, stirring occasionally. While mixture is simmering, use separate saucepan to heat remaining broth to hot; add hot broth to sauce. Add remaining ingredients except shrimp; let simmer 10 to 12 minutes; then add shrimp. Simmer 8 minutes or until shrimp are cooked. Serves 4.

   Serve each with ⅔ cup cooked rice, ½ cup cooked snap peas and 1 cup mixed melon.

Exchanges: 3 meats, 2 breads, 2 vegetables, 1 fruit, 1 fat

1 ½ lbs. shrimp, peeled and deveined
1 tbsp. canola oil
1 ½ c. chicken broth, heated
2 c. chopped onion
1 tsp. black pepper
1 c. chopped celery
1 tsp. basil leaves
⅛ tsp. cayenne pepper
   Dash red hot sauce (optional)
2 bay leaves
1 tbsp. brown sugar
2 tsp. salt
2 tsp. granulated garlic
¼ c. all-purpose flour
1 c. chopped bell pepper
2 16-oz. cans diced tomatoes
2 8-oz. cans tomato sauce

TERIYAKI BAKED FISH

Preheat oven to 450° F. Place vegetables in a microwave-safe dish and microwave according to package directions. Toss with ¼ cup teriyaki sauce. Arrange fillets in 9x9-inch dish coated with cooking spray. Bake 10 minutes per inch of thickness; remove from oven and top with remaining teriyaki sauce. Bake 2 minutes more, or until sauce is heated. While sauce is heating, toss linguine with soy sauce. Remove fillets; top with vegetables and serve over linguine. Serves 4.

   Serve each with 1 cup fresh pineapple.

Exchanges: 3 meats, 2 breads, 2 vegetables, 1 fruit

1 lb. fish fillets (snapper, tilapia or catfish)
3 c. frozen oriental-style vegetables
½ c. teriyaki sauce, divided
3 c. cooked linguine
4 tsp. soy sauce
   Nonstick cooking spray

4 oz. (about 12 medium) precooked
  shrimp
¼ c. cocktail sauce
8 saltine crackers

4 4-oz. fish fillets (snapper, catfish,
  tilapia or grouper)
  Salt and black pepper to taste
½ tsp. ground cumin
2 tsp. lime juice
  Nonstick cooking spray

4 4-oz. tuna steaks, about
  ½ in. thick
⅓ c. fresh lime juice
½ tsp. dried oregano
½ tsp. ground cumin
¼ tsp. salt
2 garlic cloves, minced
1 tsp. olive oil
1 tsp. cracked pepper
  Lime slices (optional)
  Nonstick cooking spray

SHRIMP COCKTAIL

Serve with 1 cup **Broccoli Slaw**.
Exchanges: **2 meats, 2 breads, 1 vegetable, 1 fruit, ½ fat**

SOUTHWESTERN-STYLE BAKED FISH

Preheat oven to 400° F. Coat 9x9-inch baking pan with cooking spray. Place fillets in pan; season with salt, pepper, cumin and lime juice. Bake 12 to 15 minutes (10 minutes per inch of thickness). Garnish with **Black Bean Salsa**. Serves 4.

Serve each with ⅓ cup cooked rice, a 6-inch ear of corn and 1 cup steamed broccoli topped with 1 teaspoon melted low-calorie margarine.
Exchanges: **3 meats, 2½ breads, 1½ vegetables, 1 fat**

GRILLED TUNA STEAKS

Combine lime juice, oregano, cumin, salt and garlic in large shallow dish; mix well. Add tuna; turn to coat. Cover and marinate in refrigerator 1 hour, turning steaks occasionally.

Preheat broiler. Remove tuna from dish; discard marinade. Brush oil over steaks; sprinkle with pepper. Place fish on broiler pan coated with cooking spray; broil 5 minutes or until medium—do not turn. (Cook longer to desired doneness.) Garnish with lime slices, if desired.

Serve each with ½ cup **Roasted Potatoes**, 1 cup grilled vegetables and a 1-ounce dinner roll topped with 1 teaspoon reduced-fat margarine.
Exchanges: **3 meats, 2 breads, 2 vegetables, 1 fat**

GRILLED OR BROILED HALIBUT

In 9x9-inch dish, combine dressing, Worcestershire sauce, paprika and pepper; stir to blend. Add fillets; let marinate 30 minutes in refrigerator. Preheat grill or broiler to medium-high heat. Grill fillets 10 minutes per inch of thickness, turning once.

Serve each with ½ cup **Mashed Potatoes**, 1 cup grilled assorted vegetables and a 1-ounce dinner roll.

Exchanges: 3 meats, 2 breads, 1 vegetable, ½ fat

4 4-oz. halibut fillets
2 tbsp. low-fat Italian dressing
2 tsp. Worcestershire sauce
½ tsp. paprika
¼ tsp. black pepper

SHRIMP AND VEGETABLE RISOTTO

Heat oil in large skillet. Add tomatoes, summer squash, zucchini, onion, mushrooms and garlic; sauté over medium heat until tender-crisp. Add shrimp and keep warm. In separate saucepan, combine rice, oregano and broth; bring to a boil and simmer until thickened, stirring occasionally. Stir in cheese, salt and pepper. In large bowl, combine shrimp mixture with rice mixture; toss and garnish with peas. Serves 4.

Serve each with 2 or 3 **Toasted Pita Chips**.

Exchanges: 1½ meats, 2 breads, 1½ vegetables, ½ fat

¾ lb. precooked salad shrimp
2 tbsp. olive oil
6 plum tomatoes, quartered and seeded
1 medium summer squash, cubed
1 medium zucchini, cubed
1 c. chopped onion
1 c. sliced mushrooms
1 garlic clove, minced
¾ c. uncooked Arborio rice
1 tsp. leaf oregano
3 c. chicken broth
¼ c. freshly grated Parmesan cheese
   Salt and pepper to taste
½ c. frozen peas, thawed

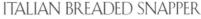

1 lb. red snapper, cut into 4 fillets
½ c. Italian-seasoned bread crumbs
½ tsp. salt
1 tbsp. fresh lemon or lime juice
1 tbsp. olive oil

ITALIAN BREADED SNAPPER

Rinse fillets; pat dry with paper towels. In shallow dish, combine bread crumbs and salt. Place lemon or lime juice in separate bowl. Dip fillets first in juice; press in bread crumbs to coat. Heat oil in large nonstick skillet; cook fillets over medium heat 4 to 5 minutes each side, turning once (about 10 minutes total for 1 inch thick fillets or until flaky when tested with fork). Serves 4.

    Serve each with ½ cup cooked pasta tossed with ¼ cup prepared marinara sauce, 1 cup steamed broccoli, a 1-ounce breadstick and 1 cup mixed berries.
Exchanges: 3 meats, 2 breads, 1 ½ vegetables, 1 fruit, ½ fat

4 4-oz. tilapia, catfish or similar
   fish fillets
¼ c. prepared Creole or brown mustard
2 tbsp. nonfat milk
1 tsp. honey
¾ c. crushed pecans (or pecan meal)
   Nonstick cooking spray

HONEY-MUSTARD PECAN TILAPIA

Preheat oven to 450° F. Rinse fillets; pat dry with paper towels. Coat baking sheet with cooking spray; set aside. Place pecans in shallow dish. In small bowl, combine mustard, milk and honey; mix well. Dip fillets in milk mixture; press into pecans to coat. Bake 12 minutes or until crisp. Serves 4.

    Serve each with ¾ cup mashed potatoes, 1 cup cooked green beans and ¾ cup mixed melon balls.
Exchanges: 3 meats, 2 breads, 1 vegetable, 1 fruit, 1 fat

2 8-oz. swordfish steaks
1 garlic clove, crushed
¼ tsp. dill weed, divided
½ tsp. dried leaf oregano, divided
¼ c. lemon juice
⅛ tsp. paprika (or to taste)
   Salt to taste (added during cooking)
   Nonstick cooking spray

GRILLED SWORDFISH WITH OREGANO

Preheat grill or broiler to medium-high. Rub steaks with garlic; place on hot grill or broiler pan coated with cooking spray. Sprinkle with half the dill, half the oregano and a little salt. Cook 4 to 5 minutes; turn and brush with lemon juice. Season with remaining dill and oregano and a little more salt. Cook additional 4 to 5 minutes or until fish is opaque throughout. Cut each in half; sprinkle with paprika. Serves 4.

    Serve each with 1 **Twice-Baked Potato** and 1 cup **Sautéed Spinach.**
Exchanges: 3 meats, 2 breads, 2 vegetables, 1 fat

GINGER AND GARLIC-BRAISED HALIBUT FILLETS

Lightly coat large nonstick skillet with cooking spray. Preheat until very hot but not smoking. Add fillets; brown skin side down for 2 minutes. Add onion, scallions, garlic, ginger and pepper flakes; cook on high 1 minute. Reduce heat; turn fillets. Add grape juice and broth; cover pan and simmer 10 minutes or until cooked through. (Insert small, thin knife into fish to check for doneness.)

While fish is simmering, prepare 4 servings instant brown rice according to package directions. Serve fish over rice and spoon some of the sauce over the fillets. Serves 4.

Serve each with ⅔ cup rice and 1 cup **Broccoli Slaw.**
Exchanges: 3 meats, 2 breads, 2 vegetables, 1 fat

1 ¼ lbs. 1 in. thick halibut fillets,
    cut into 4 pieces
1 small onion, minced
2 white scallions, chopped
2 green scallions, chopped into
    1-in. lengths
3 garlic cloves, minced
2 tbsp. minced fresh ginger
⅛ tsp. crushed red-pepper flakes
¼ c. white grape juice
½ c. canned chicken broth
2 c. uncooked instant brown rice
    Nonstick cooking spray

GINGER SALMON FILLETS

*Here's how to make a green-onion fan: Cut off the root of a green onion and then slice into the white end 2 or 3 times to create thin strips. Place in cold water for 1 hour and the onion will "fan"!

Coat broiler rack with cooking spray; preheat broiler. Combine orange juice, soy sauce, cooking sherry, ginger and honey in large zip-top plastic bag. Add fillets; seal and marinate in refrigerator 30 minutes. Remove fillets from bag and reserve marinade. Arrange fillets on broiler rack; sprinkle with salt and pepper. Broil 6 minutes or until fillets flake easily with fork, basting frequently with reserved marinade. After fillets are cooked, place remaining marinade in saucepan; bring to a boil and use as a sauce for serving. Garnish with green-onion fans, if desired. Serves 4.

Serve each with ⅔ cup **Roasted Potatoes**, 1 cup cooked green vegetables and a 1-ounce dinner roll topped with 1 teaspoon reduced-fat margarine.
Exchanges: 3 meats, 2 breads, 2 vegetables, ½ fat

4 4-oz. salmon fillets, about
    1 in. thick
¼ c. fresh orange juice
¼ c. soy sauce
¼ c. cooking sherry
¼ c. Dijon mustard
2 tbsp. grated peeled fresh ginger
2 tbsp. honey
    Green-onion fans* (optional)
    Nonstick cooking spray

3 c. cooked elbow macaroni
3 c. frozen broccoli, thawed
1 9-oz. can white tuna, packed in
   water, drained and flaked
1 8-oz. can sliced water chestnuts,
   drained
¾ c. shredded reduced-fat cheddar cheese
1 10¾-oz. can reduced-fat cream
   of mushroom soup
1 c. nonfat plain yogurt
⅓ c. nonfat dry milk powder
1 tsp. cornstarch
1 tsp. Worcestershire sauce
½ tsp. granulated garlic
¼ c. freshly grated Parmesan cheese
   Butter-flavored nonstick cooking
   spray

Preheat oven to 350° F. Spray 8x8-inch cooking dish with cooking spray. In a large bowl, combine macaroni, broccoli, tuna, water chestnuts and cheddar cheese. In separate bowl, combine soup, yogurt, milk powder, cornstarch, Worcestershire sauce and garlic. Blend well. Add soup mixture to macaroni mixture; mix well to combine. Pour into prepared casserole. Sprinkle with Parmesan cheese; cover and bake 30 minutes. Uncover and bake an additional 10 minutes. Serves 4.

Serve each with 1 cup green salad with 2 tablespoons low-fat dressing.
Exchanges: 2 meats, 2½ breads, 1 vegetable, ½ milk, 1½ fats

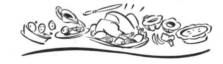

VEGETABLES AND PASTA

CHEESE LASAGNA

6 oz. uncooked whole-wheat lasagna
   noodles
½ c. tomato sauce
1 c. mixed onion, bell pepper and
   mushrooms
1½ c. low-fat cottage cheese
2 eggs
2 tbsp. freshly grated Parmesan cheese
3 oz. mozzarella cheese, grated

Cook lasagna noodles in boiling water until tender. Drain and set aside. Combine tomato sauce and chopped onion, pepper and mushrooms. In separate bowl, mix cottage cheese, eggs and ½ of the Parmesan. Preheat oven to 350°F. In an 8x8-inch casserole, layer half the noodles, the cottage cheese mixture and grated mozzarella cheese. Top with tomato sauce mix and remaining noodles; sprinkle with remaining Parmesan. Bake for 25 minutes; then serve hot. Serves 4.

Serve each with 1 cup green salad with 2 tablespoons low-fat dressing.
Exchanges: 4 meats, 2 breads, 1 fat

SPICY EGGPLANT CASSEROLE

Preheat oven to 400° F. Salt eggplants and let sit 20 minutes to draw out bitterness. Rinse and drain. In medium bowl, combine eggplants, onion, celery, bell pepper, canned tomatoes, bread cubes, salt and pepper. Pour into 9x9-inch baking dish coated with cooking spray; top with cheese and bake 20 to 25 minutes. Serves 4.

Serve each with 1 cup green salad with 2 tablespoons low-fat dressing, and a 1-ounce breadstick.

Exchanges: ½ **meat, 1 bread, 2 vegetables,** ½ **fat**

2 small eggplants, peeled and cut into
1-in. cubes
1 ½ tbsp. chopped onion
1 ½ tbsp. chopped celery
1 ½ tbsp. chopped bell pepper
1 10-oz. can diced tomatoes with chilies
½ c. soft bread cubes
Salt and cayenne pepper to taste
2 oz. 2% cheddar cheese, shredded
Nonstick cooking spray

ROASTED VEGETABLE SANDWICHES

In small bowl, combine yogurt, mayonnaise, 1 tablespoon basil and lemon juice; whisk together. (**Note:** Spread can be prepared ahead of time and refrigerated.)

Preheat oven to 450° F. In large bowl, blend vinegar, oil and basil. Add vegetables; toss to coat. Place vegetables in roasting pan and bake 30 minutes or until tender and lightly browned, stirring occasionally. Remove from oven and set aside to cool.

Spread basil-yogurt mixture over bread. Top with cheese and vegetables. Serves 4.

Exchanges: **1 meat, 2 breads, 1** ½ **vegetables, 1 fat**

8 slices sourdough bread (or 4 of either
pocket-pita breads or 2-oz. rolls)
¼ c. plain nonfat yogurt
2 tbsp. reduced-fat mayonnaise
1 tbsp. fresh basil
1 tsp. lemon juice
3 tbsp. balsamic or red wine vinegar
2 tsp. olive oil
¼ c. chopped fresh basil (or 1 tbsp.
dried)
1 small eggplant, sliced into
thin rounds
1 zucchini, thinly sliced
1 yellow summer squash, thinly sliced
1 red bell pepper, thinly sliced
1 small red onion, sliced and separated
into rings
4 oz. low-fat Swiss cheese, sliced

2 12-oz. pkgs. veggie ground round
(Yves' Light Life brand suggested)

1 15-oz. can each kidney, black and
great Northern beans

2 16-oz. cans diced tomatoes

2 large onions, chopped

2 8-oz. cans tomato sauce

2 green bell peppers, chopped

¼ tsp. paprika

2 tbsp. chili powder

2 tsp. ground cumin

6 oz. uncooked spaghetti noodles

1 tsp. vegetable oil

1 medium onion, chopped

⅔ c. reduced-sodium chicken broth

3 c. sliced mushrooms

8 oz. cooked lean Canadian bacon,
thinly sliced into strips

1 c. frozen peas

1 oz. Parmesan cheese, freshly grated

2 tbsp. reduced-fat sour cream
Freshly ground black pepper, to taste
Additional Parmesan cheese for
garnish (optional)
Nonstick cooking spray

CHILI *NON* CARNE

In large pot, combine all ingredients; stir to blend well. Bring to a boil; cover and simmer for 1 hour. Makes about 3 quarts or 8 1½-cup servings.

Serve each with 8 crackers and 1 peach.

Exchanges: **3 meats, 2½ breads, 2 vegetables, 1 fruit, ½ fat**

SPAGHETTI CARBONARA

Cook spaghetti noodles according to package directions, omitting salt and fat; drain. Return to pot; toss with oil to prevent sticking. Set aside. Coat large, non-stick skillet with cooking spray. Sauté onion over medium-high heat until tender. Add broth; bring to a boil. Add mushrooms; cook 4 to 5 minutes, stirring frequently. Add bacon strips. Cook additional 2 to 3 minutes; add peas. When heated through, remove from heat. Stir in cheese and sour cream. Garnish each serving with pepper and cheese. Serves 4.

Serve each with 1 cup salad with 2 tablespoons low-fat dressing, and a 1-ounce slice toasted French bread.

Exchanges: **2½ meats, 2½ breads, 1 vegetable, 1 fat**

VEGETABLE LASAGNA

Preheat oven to 350° F. Heat oil in saucepan. Add onion, carrots and garlic; sauté 5 to 6 minutes or until tender. Add sauce, water and spices; bring to a simmer. In small bowl, blend eggs, Ricotta and Parmesan; add vegetables. Coat 9x13-inch baking pan coated with cooking spray and spread thin layer of red sauce in bottom. Cover with a layer of noodles. Spoon half cheese-vegetable mixture over noodles; cover with half of remaining red sauce. Repeat with noodles, cheese-vegetable mixture and red sauce. Cover with foil and bake 20 minutes; remove foil and top with mozzarella. Bake uncovered 15 minutes more; let sit 10 minutes before slicing. Serves 6.

Serve each with 1 cup tossed salad with 2 tablespoons low-fat dressing, a 3-inch slice of French bread with 1 teaspoon margarine, and 1 cup **Fruit Salad**.
Exchanges: 3 meats, 2 breads, 2 vegetables, 1 fruit, 1 fat

2 tbsp. canola oil
1 c. chopped onion
1 ½ c. thinly sliced carrots
2 tsp. minced garlic
6 uncooked no-bake lasagna noodles
1 15-oz. jar spaghetti sauce
½ c. water
1 tsp. leaf basil
½ tsp. leaf oregano
2 eggs, slightly beaten
2 c. Ricotta cheese
4 tbsp. freshly shredded Parmesan cheese
1 c. sliced mushrooms
1 c. quartered and sliced zucchini
1 c. shredded part-skim mozzarella cheese
1 10-oz. pkg. frozen chopped spinach, thawed and drained
Nonstick cooking spray

SIDE DISHES

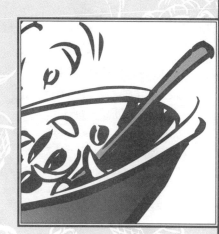

Note: To use a one-serving recipe as a multiple-serving side dish, simply multiply the ingredients depending on the number of people to be served; then serve the original measured amount to each person. The exchanges will remain the same per serving.

3 c. sweet potatoes (about 2 ½ lbs.), peeled and thinly sliced
1 small lemon, thinly sliced
2 ⅔ tbsp. orange juice
1 tsp. grated orange rind
3 ½ tbsp. firmly-packed brown sugar (or brown-sugar substitute)
2 tsp. reduced-fat margarine
  Nonstick cooking spray

3 ½ c. baking potatoes, peeled and cubed
3 garlic cloves, peeled
¼ c. 2% low-fat milk
1 tbsp. reduced-fat margarine
1 tbsp. low-fat sour cream
2 tbsp. grated Parmesan cheese
¼ tsp. salt
  Dash pepper

Side Dishes

POTATOES

ORANGE-GLAZED SWEET POTATOES

Preheat oven to 400° F. Arrange potatoes and lemon slices in 13x9-inch baking dish coated with cooking spray; set aside. Melt margarine in small bowl. Add orange juice, orange rind and brown sugar to melted margarine; mix well to blend. Drizzle mixture over potatoes; cover dish with foil. Bake 35 minutes; uncover, stir and bake 30 minutes more. Serves 4.
Exchanges: 2 breads, ½ fat

GARLIC MASHED POTATOES

Place potatoes and garlic in saucepan; cover with water. Bring to a boil; reduce heat. Simmer 20 minutes; drain and return to pan. Add milk, margarine, sour cream, Parmesan, salt and pepper. Using mixer, beat at medium speed until smooth. Serves 4.
Exchanges: 1 bread, ½ fat

TWICE-BAKED POTATOES

Preheat oven to 425° F. Pierce potatoes several times with fork; place on baking pan and bake 1 hour or until cooked through. Remove from oven; reduce temperature to 375° F. In large pot of boiling, salted water, cook broccoli 3 minutes; drain and rinse under cold water; then drain again. (Omit this step if using frozen broccoli.) Cut potatoes in half horizontally. Scoop out potatoes, leaving ½ inch of shell intact. In medium bowl, combine insides of potatoes, cheddar cheese, sour cream, milk, mustard, salt and red pepper; mix well. Gently fold in broccoli; spoon mixture evenly into potato shells; place on baking sheet and bake 10 minutes or until hot and bubbly. Serves 4.

Exchanges: 1 meat, 1 ½ breads, 1 vegetable, ½ fat
(**Note**: Omitting cheese will omit meat exchange.)

4 5-oz. russet potatoes

3 c. chopped broccoli florets (or 10 oz. frozen chopped broccoli, thawed)

4 oz. shredded reduced-fat cheddar cheese (optional)

¼ c. low-fat sour cream

¼ c. nonfat milk

1 tbsp. reduced-fat margarine

1 tsp. prepared mustard

¾ tsp. salt

⅛ tsp. ground red pepper

OVEN FRIES

Preheat oven to 450° F. Place potato sticks onto nonstick baking sheet; spray sticks lightly with nonstick cooking spray. Sprinkle with salt and paprika; bake 10 to 12 minutes or until crispy outside and tender inside. Serves 1.

Exchanges: 1 bread

1 3-oz. baking potato, cut into thin sticks

¼ tsp. salt

¼ tsp. paprika
Nonstick cooking spray

ROASTED POTATOES

Preheat oven to 450° F. In medium bowl, combine potatoes, olive oil, rosemary, pepper and Parmesan; mix well. Spoon onto 11x7-inch baking dish coated with cooking spray; bake 35 minutes or until tender, stirring occasionally. Serves 4.

Exchanges: 2 breads, ½ fat

6 red potatoes (about 1 1/2 lbs.), each cut into 8 wedges

1 tbsp. olive oil

¼ tsp. rosemary

⅛ tsp. pepper

1 tbsp. grated Parmesan cheese
Nonstick cooking spray

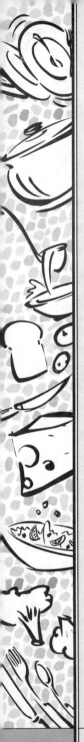

SALAD DRESSINGS

RUSSIAN DRESSING

2 ½ tsp. low-fat mayonnaise
2 ½ tsp. ketchup

Combine in small bowl and blend well. Serves 1 or 2, depending upon portion.
Exchanges: For 2 ½ teaspoons: zero exchanges
          For 1 ½ tablespoons: ½ fat

BALSAMIC VINAIGRETTE

2 tsp. balsamic vinegar
1 tsp. olive oil
   Pinch garlic powder

Combine vinegar, olive oil and garlic powder in small jar with tight-fitting lid; cover and shake well. (Can also be made in small bowl and blended with wisk.) Serves 1.
Exchanges: 1 fat

SALADS AND SLAWS

CAESAR SALAD

Combine and enjoy! Serves 1.
Exchanges: 1 vegetable, ½ bread, 12 fat

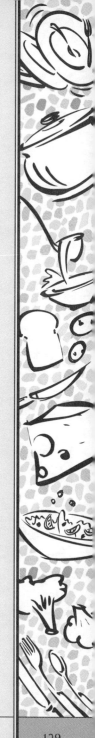

2 c. loosely packed romaine lettuce
¼ c. croutons
1 tsp. freshly grated Parmesan cheese
2 tbsp. prepared low-fat Caesar dressing (such as Ken's or Kraft)

CARROT SALAD

In large bowl, combine carrots, cabbage, pineapple and walnuts; toss well. In small bowl, combine remaining juice with mayonnaise, sugar (or substitute), vinegar and pepper; mix well. Pour dressing over slaw; toss gently to coat. Cover and refrigerate 2 to 24 hours. Serves 6.
Exchanges: 1½ vegetables, ½ fruit, 1 fat

4 c. shredded carrots
1 16-oz. can crushed pineapple, drained (reserve juice)
1 tbsp. chopped walnuts
⅓ c. low-fat mayonnaise
1 tbsp. sugar or sugar-substitute equivalent
2 tbsp. cider vinegar
½ tsp. ground black pepper

TROPICAL FRUIT SALAD

In large bowl, combine all ingredients; mix well. Chill and serve. Serves 6.
Exchanges: 1½ fruits

2 15¼-oz. cans tropical fruit salad, packed in passion-fruit nectar, drained
1 6-oz. artificially sweetened vanilla-flavored nonfat yogurt
1 tbsp. flaked coconut

1 small banana, peeled and sliced

1 navel orange, peeled and sectioned

1 c. sliced strawberries

1 c. cubed cantaloupe

1 c. cubed watermelon

½ c. blueberries

½ c. seedless grapes

1 6-oz. artificially sweetened apricot-
flavored nonfat yogurt

1 tsp. lemon juice

2 c. chopped fresh broccoli

½ c. raisins

2 tbsp. diced red onion

2 slices turkey bacon, cooked crisp

2 tbsp. plain nonfat yogurt

2 tbsp. low-fat mayonnaise

½ tbsp. cider vinegar

1 tbsp. brown sugar

1 lb. large spinach, leaves removed

2 tsp. sesame oil

1 tsp. soy sauce

1 tsp. salt

2 tsp. sesame seeds

FRUIT SALAD

In large bowl combine all ingredients; toss well. Serves 4.
Exchanges: 1½ fruits

BROCCOLI SALAD

Blanch broccoli in boiling water; drain and rinse with cold water to stop cooking process. In medium bowl, combine broccoli, raisins, onion and bacon; set aside. Combine yogurt, mayonnaise, vinegar and brown sugar in small bowl; mix well and pour onto broccoli mixture. Toss to coat; chill at least 2 hours. Serves 4.
Exchanges: 1 vegetable, 1 fruit, 1 fat

SESAME SPINACH SALAD

Blanch spinach for 1 minute in boiling water; drain and squeeze dry. In large bowl, combine sesame oil, soy sauce, salt and sesame seeds; mix well. Add spinach and toss to coat. Serves 4.
Exchanges: 1 vegetable, 1 fat

POTATO SALAD

Place potatoes in a large saucepan; cover with water and bring to a boil. Cook 8 minutes or until tender. Drain; place in large bowl. Add onion, celery, relish, egg and garlic; toss gently and set aside. In medium bowl, combine sour cream, mayonnaise, mustard, salt and pepper; stir well. Pour over potato mixture; toss gently to coat. Cover and chill. Serves 6.
Exchanges: 1 bread, ½ fat

4 c. (about 1 ½ lbs.) cubed, unpeeled red potatoes
¼ c. diced onion
¼ c. diced celery
⅛ c. drained sweet- or dill-pickle relish
1 hard-boiled egg, chopped
½ garlic clove, minced
¼ c. low-fat sour cream
¼ c. low-fat mayonnaise
½ tsp. dry mustard
¼ tsp. salt
⅛ tsp. pepper

MIXED BEAN SALAD

Combine all ingredients in medium bowl; refrigerate covered at least 1 hour. Serves 1.
Exchanges: 1 ½ vegetables, ½ fat

⅓ c. steamed green beans, cooled
⅓ c. wax beans
⅓ c. sugar snap peas
2 tbsp. low-fat Italian dressing

PICKLED BEET AND ONION SALAD

Combine all ingredients in medium bowl; refrigerate, covered, at least 1 hour. Serves 1.
Exchanges: 1 vegetable

1 c. sliced cooked beets
½ c. sliced onion
2 tbsp. cider vinegar
1 tsp. canola oil
Sugar substitute to equal
2 tsp. sugar
Freshly ground black pepper, to taste

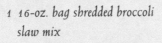

1 16-oz. bag shredded broccoli
   slaw mix
¼ c. sweet pickle relish
⅓ c. low-fat mayonnaise
1 tsp. prepared brown mustard
¼ tsp. celery seed
¼ tsp. black pepper
1 c. (about 15) red grapes (optional)

1 medium head Savoy cabbage,
   untrimmed
½ c. coarsely shredded red cabbage
½ c. corn kernels
½ oz. low-fat cheddar cheese, shredded
⅓ c. chunky salsa
2 tbsp. plain nonfat yogurt
2 tsp. fat-free sour cream
¼ tsp. chili powder

2 tbsp. low-fat mayonnaise
1 tbsp. plain nonfat yogurt
1 tsp. cider vinegar
1 tsp. sugar
¼ tsp. paprika
3 c. finely shredded cabbage
1 c. chopped carrots
¼ c. diced onion
¼ c. diced bell pepper
   Salt and pepper to taste

BROCCOLI SLAW

Combine all ingredients in large bowl; refrigerate until needed. Serves 4.
Exchanges: 1 vegetable

SOUTHWESTERN COLESLAW

Remove 4 outer leaves from Savoy cabbage; set aside. Coarsely shred inner leaves; combine with red cabbage, corn and cheddar cheese in large bowl; set aside. In small bowl, combine salsa, yogurt, sour cream and chili powder; blend well. Add dressing to cabbage mixture, tossing gently. Cover and chill. Serve in reserved leaves. Serves 4.
Exchanges: 1 vegetable

SUMMER COLESLAW

In large bowl, combine mayonnaise, yogurt, vinegar, sugar and paprika; mix well. Add cabbage, carrots, onion and bell pepper; stir to blend and season with salt and pepper. Refrigerate at least 1 hour. Serves 4.
Exchanges: 1½ vegetables, ½ fat

MARINATED CUCUMBERS

Using fork to score cucumber down its side. Thinly slice and discard ends. In glass bowl or dish, combine cucumber, onion, pepper and dressing. Marinate at least 2 hours; then drain liquid and serve on spinach leaves. Serves 4.
Exchange: 1 vegetable, ½ fat

2 large cucumbers
½ c. sliced sweet onion (Vidalia, Texas Sweet or Walla Walla)
¼ tsp. black pepper
⅓ c. low-fat Italian dressing
   Spinach leaves for garnish

ITALIAN HERBED TOMATOES

Arrange tomatoes in shallow bowl; set aside. Use small bowl to combine olive oil, vinegar, Italian seasoning, garlic powder and pepper; mix well and pour over tomatoes. Marinate at least 30 minutes before serving. Serves 2.
Exchange: 1 vegetable, ½ fat

2 c. sliced tomatoes
1 tsp. olive oil
2 tbsp. balsamic vinegar
¼ tsp. Italian seasoning
⅛ tsp. garlic powder
⅛ tsp. black pepper

SALSAS

CORN SALSA

1 ½ c. frozen corn kernels, thawed
¼ c. chopped red onion
¼ c. chopped red bell pepper
¼ c. chopped fresh cilantro
1 ½ tbsp. fresh lime juice
1 to 2 tsp. seeded chopped jalapeño peppers
Salt and pepper to taste

(**Note:** Salsa may be made the day before using; then cover and refrigerate until needed.)
Combine all ingredients in large bowl; refrigerate until needed. Makes 4 servings.
Exchanges: 1 bread

BLACK BEAN SALSA

1 16-oz. can black beans, drained
1 c. chunky salsa
1 tbsp. diced red onion
1 tbsp. chopped fresh cilantro
1 tsp. chili powder

(**Note:** Salsa may be made the day before using; then cover and refrigerate until needed.)
Combine all ingredients in large bowl; refrigerate until needed. Serves 4.
Exchanges: 1 bread, ½ vegetable

THIS 'N' THAT

CORNBREAD

Preheat oven to 425° F. In 9-inch cast-iron skillet melt margarine over medium heat. Combine flour, cornmeal, baking powder and salt in large bowl; add buttermilk and egg, stirring just until moist. Pour batter into skillet; bake 25 to 30 minutes or until a wooden pick inserted in center comes out clean. Serves 12.
Exchanges: 1 bread, ½ fat

2 tbsp. margarine
1 c. all-purpose flour
1 c. yellow cornmeal
2 ½ tsp. baking powder
½ tsp. salt
1 c. buttermilk
1 large egg, lightly beaten

MARINARA SAUCE

Purée tomatoes in blender or food processor. Heat oil in medium saucepan over medium-high heat. Add garlic; sauté 15 seconds, stirring constantly (do not let brown). Add tomato purée, tomato paste, oregano, red-pepper flakes, salt and pepper. Bring sauce to boil; reduce heat and simmer 20 minutes. Remove from heat; stir in parsley. Serves 5.
Exchanges: 2 vegetables, ½ fat
(**Note:** Serving sauce over 2 cups cooked linguini adds 2 bread exchanges.)

2 16-oz. cans peeled plum tomatoes
2 tsp. olive oil
5 tsp. finely minced garlic
1 6-oz. can tomato paste
1 ½ tsp. dried oregano, crumbled
½ tsp. red-pepper flakes
Salt and pepper, to taste
⅔ c. fresh parsley, minced

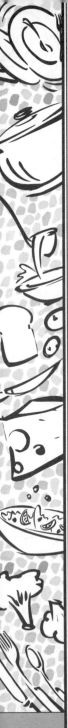

1 c. packaged cornflake crumbs
¼ tsp. granulated garlic
1 tsp. paprika
¼ tsp. onion powder
1 tsp. instant chicken bouillon
⅛ tsp. black pepper
½ tsp. poultry seasoning

2½ c. cooked elbow macaroni (about
    12 oz. uncooked)
3 tbsp. all-purpose flour
1 c. 1% low-fat milk
⅓ c. shredded sharp cheddar cheese
⅓ c. freshly grated Parmesan cheese,
    divided
    Dash paprika
    Dash salt
    Dash freshly ground pepper
    Nonstick cooking spray

2 6-in. pita bread pockets
¼ tsp. garlic salt
    Butter-flavored nonstick
    cooking spray

ALL-PURPOSE BREADING MIX

Combine all ingredients and mix well. Store in an airtight container; mix well before using. Makes about 1 cup. Plan on using 2 tablespoons for each chicken breast (you can substitute fish fillet for chicken).
Exchanges: 2 tablespoons = ½ bread

MACARONI AND CHEESE

Preheat oven to 350° F. Place flour in large saucepan. Gradually add milk, stirring constantly with whisk to blend. Cook over medium heat 8 minutes or until thick, stirring constantly. Add all of cheddar, ½ cup Parmesan, salt and pepper; cook 3 minutes or until cheese melts, stirring frequently. Remove from heat; stir in macaroni. Pour into baking dish coated with cooking spray; bake 10 minutes. Serves 4.
Exchanges: 1½ meats, 2 breads, 1 fat

TOASTED PITA CHIPS

(**Note:** These are great with dips, in soups and with lunches. For more fiber, use whole-wheat pita bread.)
Preheat oven to 325° F. Split each pita pocket in half with a sharp knife; cut each half into 6 triangles (24 total). Arrange triangles in single layers on cookie sheets; coat with cooking spray and sprinkle lightly with garlic salt. Bake for 8 minutes or until chips are lightly browned and very crisp. Store in airtight container until ready to serve. Serves 4.
Exchanges: 1 bread

RICE PILAF

Preheat oil in medium saucepan over medium-high heat. Add onion and garlic; sauté 2 minutes. Add broth, salt and pepper. Bring to boil; add rice. Cover and reduce heat; simmer 35 minutes. Remove from heat; let stand 5 minutes. Stir in chives, green onions and mushrooms. Serves 4.

Exchanges: 1 ½ breads, ½ vegetable, ½ fat

2 tsp. olive oil
½ c. minced fresh onion
1 garlic clove, minced
2 c. low-salt chicken broth
½ tsp. salt
½ tsp. white pepper
¾ c. uncooked long-grain rice
2 tbsp. chopped chives
¼ c. thinly sliced green onions
1 8-oz. pkg. mushrooms, chopped

REDUCED-FAT ALFREDO SAUCE

In medium saucepan, combine milk, half-and-half and butter. Cook over medium heat until butter melts and mixture is hot. Gradually stir in Parmesan cheese and garlic; stir until cheese is melted. Remove from heat; add sour cream, chives and pepper to taste. Serves 4.

Exchanges: ½ meat, ½ milk, 1 fat
(**Note:** Serving sauce over 2 cups cooked fettuccini adds 2 bread exchanges.)

¾ c. evaporated nonfat milk
¼ c. half-and-half
1 tbsp. butter, cut into 3 small pieces
½ c. freshly grated Parmesan cheese
½ tsp. garlic salt
¼ c. fat-free sour cream
2 tbsp. snipped fresh chives
Freshly ground black pepper, to taste

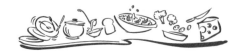

VEGGIES

CREOLE GREEN BEANS

1 lb. fresh green beans
½ small onion, diced
1 tsp. vegetable oil
1 14-oz. can seasoned diced tomatoes, with liquid
½ tsp. salt
¼ tsp. black pepper

Trim and cut green beans into 2-inch pieces. Cook in water until just tender and drain. In a large skillet, sauté onion in oil for 2 minutes. Add cooked green beans, tomatoes, salt and pepper; simmer uncovered 5 minutes. Serve hot. Serves 4.
Exchanges: 2 vegetables

MARINATED GREEN BEANS

1 lb. fresh green beans
½ small red onion, diced
1 tbsp. diced pimientos
½ c. balsamic vinegar
1 tbsp. olive oil
1 tbsp. water
½ tsp. garlic salt
¼ tsp. black pepper

Trim and cut green beans into 2-inch pieces. Cook in water until just tender; drain and place in large bowl. Add onion, pimientos, vinegar, olive oil, water, garlic salt and pepper; toss to coat; cover and refrigerate overnight. Serves 4.
Exchanges: 2 vegetables, ½ fat

BAKED ZUCCHINI

2½ lbs. small zucchini
1 tsp. olive or vegetable oil
¼ tsp. salt
⅛ tsp. freshly ground black pepper

Preheat oven to 450° F. Cut off ends and slice zucchini in half crosswise; cut each half lengthwise into quarters. In large bowl, toss zucchini with oil, salt and pepper. Arrange zucchini on jelly-roll pan in a single layer. Bake 30 minutes or until tender; transfer to serving bowl. Serves 4.
Exchanges: 1 vegetable

BRAISED CABBAGE

Generously spray skillet or Dutch oven with cooking spray. Heat and braise cabbage and onions. When tender, add a few drops of soy sauce and sprinkle with black pepper to taste. (May substitute cabbage with other greens such as turnip, kale or collards.) Serves 4.

Exchange: 1 vegetable

4 c. raw cabbage
¼ c. green onions
Soy sauce, to taste
Black pepper, to taste
Butter-flavored nonstick cooking spray

SAUTÉED SQUASH WITH PEPPERS

Cut off ends and slice squash ¼-inch thick; place in bowl and set aside. Heat butter and oil in large skillet. Add onion and bell pepper; sauté until limp. Add squash, salt and pepper; stir to mix thoroughly. Sauté over medium-high heat 3 to 4 minutes or until squash is tender. Serves 4.

Exchanges: 1 vegetable, ½ fat

1 lb. crookneck squash
2 tsp. reduced-fat butter
1 tsp. olive oil
1 tbsp. finely chopped onion
1 small green bell pepper, diced
1 tsp. salt
½ tsp. black pepper

SAUTÉED SPINACH

Trim stems from spinach; soak well in copious amounts of cool water to wash away sand. Shake water from greens and dry with paper towels. (**Note:** Spinach must be as dry as possible before cooking.) Preheat oil in heavy, wide sauté pan; add garlic. Stir; immediately add spinach (all at once if possible). Continue stirring 5 minutes; season with salt and vinegar. Serve immediately. Serves 4.

Exchanges: 1½ vegetables, ½ fat

1 lb. fresh spinach leaves
¾ tbsp. olive oil
2 tsp. chopped garlic
½ tsp. salt
Splash cider vinegar

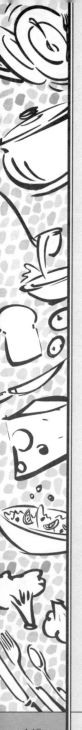

SAUTÉED SUGAR SNAP PEAS

1 tsp. olive oil
1 16-oz. pkg. frozen sugar snap
    peas, thawed
½ c. chopped onion
½ c. sliced mushrooms
    Salt and pepper to taste

Preheat olive oil in large skillet over medium-high heat. Sauté onion and mush-rooms until tender; add peas and sauté 3 to 4 minutes more. Season with salt and pepper. Serves 4.
Exchange: 2 vegetables

SAUTÉED ORIENTAL VEGETABLES

1 16-oz. pkg. frozen oriental-style
    vegetables, thawed
1 tbsp. olive oil
2 tbsp. teriyaki baste-and-glaze sauce
½ tsp. ground ginger
½ tsp. granulated garlic
1 tbsp. water, if needed

In a large skillet, sauté vegetables in olive oil until tender-crisp. Stir in teriyaki sauce, ginger and garlic, stirring constantly for 2 minutes. Thin with water if needed. Serve hot. Serves 4.
Exchanges: 1½ vegetables, ½ fat

CREOLE ZUCCHINI

1 tbsp. reduced-fat margarine
1 small onion, chopped
½ c. sliced celery
⅛ tsp. garlic powder
⅛ tsp. leaf oregano
    Dash black pepper
2 c. sliced zucchini
1 16-oz. can diced tomatoes
    with herbs

Melt margarine in medium nonstick skillet; sauté onion, celery, garlic powder, oregano and pepper. Add zucchini and tomatoes; simmer covered 30 minutes. Serves 4.
Exchanges: 1½ vegetables, ½ fat

STEWED OKRA AND TOMATOES

Combine okra, onions, tomatoes and margarine in nonstick skillet. Add salt and pepper to taste; simmer over medium heat 20 minutes or until okra is tender. Serves 4.
Exchanges: 1 ½ vegetables, ½ fat

1 10-oz. pkg. frozen cut okra
⅓ c. chopped onion
1 16-oz. can diced tomatoes
 with herbs
1 tbsp. reduced-fat margarine
 Salt and pepper to taste

VEGETABLE MEDLEY

Preheat oil to medium heat in large skillet or Dutch oven. Add squash, zucchini, carrots, onion, mushrooms, celery, cabbage and garlic powder. Cover and cook over medium heat 5 minutes, stirring occasionally. Add tomatoes, soy sauce and pepper (and any other herb you'd like). Cook 2 to 3 minutes more or until heated through. Serve immediately. Serves 4.
Exchanges: 1 vegetable, ½ fat

1 tbsp. vegetable oil
½ c. thinly sliced yellow squash
½ c. thinly sliced zucchini
½ c. diagonally sliced carrots
¼ c. chopped onion
½ c. sliced mushrooms
½ c. diagonally sliced celery
1 c. thinly sliced cabbage or bok choy
½ tsp. garlic powder
8 cherry tomatoes, halved
 Soy sauce, to taste
 Dash pepper

GRILLED EGGPLANT

Cut eggplant into ¾-inch thick slices. Sprinkle with salt; let set 10 minutes to remove bitterness. Rinse and pat dry with paper towels. Coat both sides of each slice with olive oil; then spray with cooking spray. Sprinkle one side with ½ the oregano and garlic powder; cook 4 minutes on preheated medium-hot grill or skillet. Flip and sprinkle with remaining oregano and garlic; cook 2 to 3 minutes more. Serve hot, sprinkled with Parmesan cheese. Serves 4.
Exchange: 1 vegetable

1 medium eggplant, peeled
1 tsp. salt
1 tsp. olive oil
¼ tsp. leaf oregano, divided
¼ tsp. garlic powder, divided
1 tbsp. freshly grated Parmesan cheese
 Butter-flavored nonstick cooking
 spray

1 16-oz. can Italian cut green beans,
   drained and rinsed
1 tomato, chopped
½ green bell pepper, chopped
⅓ c. sliced green onions
¼ tsp. garlic powder
¼ tsp. leaf basil
⅛ tsp. dried rosemary
   Dash black pepper

1 c. cauliflower pieces (bite sized)
1 c. broccoli pieces (bite sized)
½ c. sliced celery, cut into bite-sized
   pieces
⅓ c. chopped red onion
1 c. mushroom caps
¾ c. sliced carrots
⅓ c. cherry-tomato halves
1 tbsp. lemon juice
¼ tsp. dried dill weed
2 tbsp. low-fat ranch dressing
   Butter-flavored nonstick cooking
   spray

ITALIAN GREEN BEANS

Combine green beans, tomato, bell pepper, onion, garlic powder, basil, rosemary and pepper in microwave-safe dish. Cover and heat 3 minutes on high. Stir and rotate; heat 2 minutes more. Serves 4.
Exchange: 2 vegetables

OVEN-ROASTED VEGETABLES

Preheat oven to 400° F. In large bowl, combine cauliflower, broccoli, celery, onion, carrots, mushrooms and tomatoes; toss to mix. Arrange vegetables on baking pan coated with cooking spray. Spray vegetables lightly with cooking spray; bake 20 minutes or until tender.

While vegetables are cooking, use same bowl to combine lemon juice, dill weed and dressing; mix well and set aside. Remove vegetables from oven; drain and return to bowl. Toss to coat; serve hot. Serves 4.
Exchange: 2 vegetables

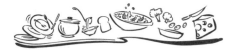

FREE FOODS

Here's one area where you can have all you want (when prepared without added fat). One exchange is for a serving size of 1 cup raw or ½ cup cooked.

The following may be steamed, broiled, sautéed, braised or grilled alone or in any combination. Be creative but, more importantly, choose a variety so that you get all of the vitamins and nutrients that you need. The variety will also keep you interested and you will tend to eat more of this good choice.

Asparagus	Green Beans
Bok Choy	Mushrooms
Broccoli	Okra
Brussels Sprouts	Onion
Cabbage	Peppers
Carrots	Snap Peas
Cauliflower	Spinach
Celery	Summer Squash
Cucumbers	Tomatoes
Eggplant	Zucchini

HEALTHY LIVING

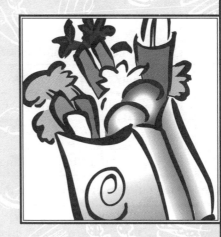

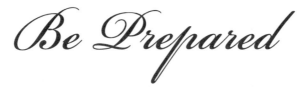

Be Prepared

SUPERMARKET GUIDE:
SOLUTIONS FOR HEALTHY SHOPPING

Do you realize that some of the most important health decisions you make are in the supermarket? That's right, healthy nutrition begins in the aisles of your grocery store! How do you decide what to buy when you shop?

	Yes	No
Do you purchase certain foods out of habit?		
Do you buy foods for taste or convenience?		
Do you usually choose those brands that are most familiar to you?		
Do you look for what's on sale or use coupons to help you decide?		
Do you read nutrition labels and comparison shop to help you choose the healthiest foods?		
Are you overwhelmed by the thousands of choices in the aisles of your grocery store?		

No matter how you answered these questions, you can use this helpful shopping guide and your nutrition knowledge to choose those foods that will help you reach your goals for a healthy weight and good overall health.

MAKING A PLAN

The best way to buy those foods that fit into your eating plan is to *plan ahead*. Before you go to the store:

Plan for Several Days at a Time

- What dishes will you be preparing?
- What foods will you need for breakfast, lunch and dinner?
- Will you be eating out during the week?
- Planning ahead will eliminate the wasted time of having to make a second or third trip to the store.

Check Cupboards, Refrigerator and Freezer
- Take stock of what you have, so you can use these foods first in upcoming meals.
- As you look, begin making a list of things you need from the store.

Prepare a List
- Keep an ongoing list in a convenient place in your kitchen.
- Add foods, supplies and ingredients to your list as you think of them.
- Use coupons only for food that fits into your eating plan.
- Before you go shopping, compare your grocery list with your meal plan to make sure you have listed all the things you need.

Before You Leave
- Eat before you shop; never go to the store on an empty stomach!
- Plan on shopping during off-hours: early in the morning, late in the evening and midweek. When it's less crowded, you'll be more relaxed and have more time to make healthy decisions.
- Lace up your walking shoes so you can pick up the pace as you shop—every bit of physical activity counts! Plan on parking a little further away from the store entrance.

At the Store
- Rely on your list to help you stick to your shopping plan.
- First, walk around the outside aisles of your store. That's where you'll find the fresh produce, dairy products, baked goods, fresh meats, poultry and fish. Save the inside aisles, which contain more processed foods, for last.
- When it comes to shopping, try not to bring home foods that don't fit into your eating plan.
- Use food labels to help you make the healthiest choices.

Beef fat	Coconut oil	Lard
Butter	Hardened shortening	Palm kernel oil
Chicken fat	Hydrogenated shortening	Palm oil

STOCKING THE HEALTHY KITCHEN

 Deciding you want to eat more healthfully is easy. It's much more difficult to actually make it happen! This can be particularly challenging for meals prepared at home. How many times have your intentions been good, but there just wasn't anything good to fix for dinner? If healthy food choices aren't kept in the kitchen, then the battle is lost before it's begun.

It is essential that your kitchen shelves reflect the new food goals you have set for yourself. Does this mean purchasing all fat-free, sugar-free and no-taste foods? Of course not! It does mean keeping certain foods on hand to provide you with lots of healthy choices. There are several things to consider as you begin planning your healthy kitchen.

FOODS YOU WILL REALLY EAT

Don't purchase foods because you *think* you should eat them. Purchase foods you *know* you'll eat. If rice cakes don't really suit your taste buds, don't buy them. Low-fat animal crackers or graham crackers may be more to your liking, so keep those on hand instead. You'll have to experiment a little to find what healthy foods you like best.

FREQUENCY OF USE

This is particularly important for cooking oils, flours, snack items, meat and fresh fruits and vegetables. Some foods might be used in small amounts—such as olive oil—and will last a long time. Buying in smaller quantities allows for greater freshness and less waste. Some foods tend to dry out and become stale quickly. It is better to buy single-serving sizes and enjoy all of them than to eat a few and throw out the rest. Using canned and frozen fruits and vegetables are great choices, especially if you find your fresh versions are always spoiling before you eat them. Freezing breads and flours is a good way to preserve their freshness.

PREPARATION TIME

For most people, time is a big consideration when planning a meal. Having a refrigerator stocked full of fresh produce and lean meat looks great, but if there isn't time to cook, it usually just ends up in the trash. Anticipate having a few times when you won't have time to cook. Keep some low-fat convenience foods on hand so you're not caught unprepared. Cooking extra and freezing the leftovers in single servings is a great way to have your own fast food!

LIST MAKING

After seriously considering your needs and preferences, go ahead and make out a kitchen list. Start by making a list of what you *normally* buy—no special foods or changes. Review your list to see if there are some items that you're willing to make healthy substitutions for. For example, you may be willing to substitute nonfat milk for 2% milk. Maybe the fried tortilla chips could be traded for baked chips or pretzels. You should also make a list of new foods you're willing to try. Use the following chart to help you:

BASIC ITEMS TO KEEP ON HAND

In the Refrigerator

Eggs	Eggs are a great source of lean protein, as well as a common ingredient for most baking. Learn to cook with egg whites and leave the yolk behind. Egg substitutes are also fine.
Milk	Keep plenty of low-fat (1%) or nonfat milk on hand; it's a great source of calcium.
Cheese	Reduced-fat or low-fat cheeses are your best choices. When you only have time for quick meal, a slice of cheese and whole-grain bread is a healthy choice. Grated cheese allows you to use less for the same amount of flavor. Choose sharp flavors.
Lunch meats	Keep a low-fat variety such as turkey or chicken breast on hand. Be sure to purchase in quantities that you actually eat! Try to choose low-sodium versions.
Salad in a bag	It's washed and ready to go! Use nonfat or low-fat dressing.
Salad dressing	Choose "light," "low-fat," "reduced-fat," "nonfat" or "low-calorie" varieties; you may have to experiment to find one or two favorites.
Fruits and vegetables	Make a list of your favorites and stock up every time you go to the store. Buy only what you can eat in one week. Cut up your vegetables when you first get home from the store so they're ready to go. Juices are also a good choice when you're on the run.

In the Freezer

Frozen vegetables	Buy in bags instead of boxes; allows you to use only what you need. You can buy individual servings too.
Frozen entrées	Choose entrées with 200 to 300 calories, 10 or fewer grams of fat and 400 or fewer milligrams of sodium.
Snacks	Choose low-calorie items such as fruit bars or sherbet.

In the Pantry

Oils	Choose at least one monounsaturated oil—olive or canola—and one polyunsaturated oil: corn, safflower or sunflower. Purchase only the amount you'll use over a few months, so it doesn't go bad before you use it.
Nonstick spray	Essential for low-fat cooking. Specialty stores sell spray bottles to make your own.
Canned foods	Keep canned vegetables such as corn, green beans, canned tomatoes, etc. These are commonly used items in casseroles and soups. Look for low-sodium varieties.
Pasta	Always have a package of pasta ready to use! Choose a prepared pasta sauce that's low in fat. Prepackaged pasta dishes can be high in fat and sodium.
Rice	Add rice to a variety of meals. You may want to have two or three varieties, such as wild rice, basmati and your favorite flavored rice, but watch out for sodium.
Cereal	Keep plenty of low-fat cereal around. Good choices are shredded wheat, bran cereals and oatmeal.
Breakfast foods	Low-fat toaster pastries or granola bars for those grab-and-go mornings.
Snacks	Choose only healthy snack foods: popcorn, low-fat cookies, low-fat snack crackers, rice cakes, dried fruits, etc. You can't eat what's not in the house!
Herbs and spices	Make sure you have lots of herbs and spices on hand. Don't be afraid to try new ones! Keep a list of your favorites; replace them after about one year.

Of course, this is not an exhaustive list, but it should get you headed in the right direction. With time you will discover the items you need in your kitchen for healthy eating. The trick is to stock a kitchen that works best for you and provides a variety of healthy foods to choose from any time.

TOOLS FOR A HEALTHY KITCHEN

Food choices and cooking methods are changing rapidly. Most of the recent changes reflect the desire of Americans to improve their health through better nutrition. Is your kitchen ready for this new way of cooking? While eating healthy doesn't require you to invest a lot of money in your kitchen, it's important to have the right equipment to get the job done. By keeping a few simple appliances and utensils handy, you'll be ready to cook healthy any time. Having the right tools saves time and allows you to focus on other important things in life.

Having the right appliances, pots and pans, cooking utensils and storage containers can help you when cooking the healthy way. Start by surveying your kitchen to see what you have on hand.

Baking dishes and pans	Do you have the variety of shapes and sizes you need?
Blender	A blender can be used to purée, grate, chop and blend. It's also great for making healthy smoothies—a frozen fruit and dairy drink.
Cheese grater	Grating cheese allows you to use less—for the same amount of flavor. You can also use it for vegetables.
Egg separator	The egg yolk contains the fat and cholesterol. You can use only the egg whites in several recipes without affecting taste or texture.
Food processor	This machine allows you to purée, grate, chop and blend foods quickly.
Freezer bags	A great way to store leftovers. Keeping lots of different sizes on hand allows you to store large or small portions. Freezing in individual serving sizes provides quick meals that need little reheating time.
Gravy separator	Allows you to separate, or remove, unwanted fat from liquids. A kitchen syringe (meat baster) can also do the trick.

Herb and spice rack	Make flavorful seasonings convenient to use and store.
Hot-air popcorn popper	Requires no butter or oil. Add your own low-fat, no-salt seasonings.
Indoor/outdoor grill	Grilling allows the fat to drip freely from the meat.
Kitchen scale	This item is especially important when trying to determine portion sizes for foods such as meats, fish, chicken or cheese.
Kitchen scissors	Probably the easiest and quickest way to trim visible fat. Use your kitchen scissors only for food!
Measuring cups/ spoons	Make sure you have plenty, so you can work with both wet and dry ingredients. The only way to learn about portion sizes is to measure everything you eat.
Meat thermometer	Takes the guesswork out of cooking meats and improves food safety.
Microwave	You probably have a microwave, but do you know how to take full advantage of all it can do?
Nonstick pots and pans	Make sure you have an assortment of nonstick pots and pans.
Nonstick skillet	This allows you to cook without adding fat. It also makes for easier cleanup!
Pastry brush	Perfect for when you need to put a light coat of oil on foods before cooking.
Plastic containers	These are great for the refrigerator. Clear containers let you see what is in them, so you are less likely to forget about leftovers. Some containers can go in the freezer as well as the microwave.
Plastic cutting board	Make sure you have a clean and safe surface for cutting and chopping. Clean your cutting board after every use with hot soapy water.
Roasting/broiling pan	Great for cooking meat the low-fat way—allows you to leave the fat behind.
Sharp knives	A good set of knives is indispensable to healthy and safe food preparation. Keep your knives sharpened and stored in a safe place.

Slotted spoon	Allows you to leave the fat and liquid behind.
Steamer	Steaming is a great way to cook vegetables, rice, poultry and fish.
Strainer or colander	Use it to strain and rinse the sodium from canned meats, legumes and vegetables. Use it to thaw frozen fruits and vegetables under running water. A microwave-safe strainer can be used to cook meats and collect fat drippings underneath.
Wok	A wok is a fast and easy way to prepare vegetables and stir-fry recipes. Most woks come with a nonstick surface, which allows you to use less oil (or no oil).

If your budget is tight, many of these will make terrific gifts for birthdays and holidays. If you don't have what you need to cook at home, are you more likely to eat out? Investing in the right tools saves money in the long run.

Organizing Your Kitchen

Not only is it important to have the tools you need, it's important to be organized.

- Keep your kitchen counter space clean and clear of junk (e.g., mail, newspapers, magazines and whatever else might be lying around).
- Organize pots, pans and other cooking utensils for easy use and storage.
- Clean dishes as you cook, which saves time in the long run.
- Assemble all ingredients and utensils in one place. Make sure you have everything you need before you start to cook.

Be Informed

UNDERSTANDING THE NUTRITION FACTS PANEL

You don't need a degree in nutrition or chemistry to eat healthy. The nutrition facts panel gives you all you need to know. Learning to read labels can help you choose the foods that best fit into your Live-It plan. The nutrition facts panel provides information on calories, fat, saturated fat, cholesterol, fiber and other important nutrients in a single serving. The ingredients list tells you what's in a food, with ingredients listed from most to least. Food labels can also include nutrition and health claims.

SERVING SIZE

The serving size is based on a typical portion, not necessarily the recommended serving. Compare the serving size on the panel with the exchange for that food. Is it more or less? How does the serving size compare to what you eat? Controlling serving size is the best way to make your Live-It plan work for you.

PERCENT DAILY VALUE

The Percent Daily Value, or % Daily Value, shows how one serving counts toward the recommended daily intake for specific nutrients. The percentage is based on a 2,000-calorie diet. Use the Percent Daily Value to see if a food is high or low in specific nutrients.

CALORIES

How does the calorie level compare to what you know about the calorie exchange for that food? Calories from fat are indicated by the *number* of calories from fat, *not* the percentage. If you want to determine the percentage, divide the calories from fat by the calories. On average, choose more foods with 30 percent or less of calories from fat. Not every food you eat has to be less than 30 percent fat—just the overall balance of foods you eat!

HEALTHY LIVING

NUTRIENTS

Total fat, saturated fat, cholesterol, sodium, carbohydrates, fiber, sugars, protein, vitamins A and C, calcium and iron must be listed on the label. Vitamins and minerals added to foods must also be listed.

For total fat, saturated fat, cholesterol and sodium, look for foods with a low percent daily value.

For vitamins, minerals and fiber, your goal is to reach 100 percent each day. Choose foods with a high percentage of nutrients; a good source contains 10 percent or more.

At the bottom of the panel is the recommended amount of important nutrients for a 2,000 and a 2,500 calorie diet. It shows the maximum amounts of total fat, saturated fat, cholesterol and sodium recommended for a healthy and balanced eating plan: no more than 30 percent calories from fat, less than 10 percent saturated fat and less than 60 percent of total calories from carbohydrates. The last item on the panel is the number of calories per gram of fat, carbohydrate and protein.

> **A note about sodium:** Although there is currently no Recommended Daily Intake (RDI)[1] for sodium, it is an electrolyte that is necessary for good health. Experts estimate that the body needs about 500 milligrams per day to maintain fluid balance, help muscles contract, aid in nerve transmissions and even regulate blood pressure. Most guidelines recommend that daily sodium consumption be limited to 2,400 for fewer milligrams, or 1 teaspoon of table salt, per day.[2] This amount is far less than the 4,000 to 6,000 milligrams consumed by the average American.

USING THE LABEL TO FIGURE OUT EXCHANGES

The nutrition facts panel gives you all you need to know to figure out the exchanges for a typical serving of any food: total calories and grams of fat, protein and carbohydrate. Be sure to adjust the calorie and nutrient amounts if you're eating more or less than one serving. Some food labels even provide the exchanges. If not, you can call the manufacturer or distributor and ask for the exchanges for that food. Most labels list the phone number and address you can call for information.

UNDERSTANDING NUTRITION AND HEALTH CLAIMS

When it comes to health and nutrition claims, you can believe what you read. Food makers must meet strict government guidelines to list terms such as "low fat" or "reduced sodium" or to make health claims about heart disease, cancer or other diseases. Only health claims that are supported by scientific evidence and approved by the Food and Drug Administration (FDA) are allowed.

Understanding Terms

Calorie free	5 calories or fewer per serving
Low calorie	40 or fewer calories per serving
Fat free	Less than $\frac{1}{2}$ (0.5) gram of total fat per serving
Low fat	3 or fewer grams of total fat per serving
Saturated fat free	Less than $\frac{1}{2}$ gram of saturated fat per serving
Low saturated fat	Less than 1 gram of saturated fat per serving
Cholesterol free	2 milligrams or fewer of cholesterol and 2 or fewer grams of saturated fat per serving
Low cholesterol	20 or fewer milligrams of cholesterol and 2 or fewer grams of saturated fat per serving
Sodium free	5 or fewer milligrams of sodium per serving
Low sodium	140 or fewer milligrams of sodium per serving
Very low sodium	35 or fewer milligrams of sodium per serving
Sugar free	Less than 0.5 gram of sugar per serving
No sugar added	No sugars added during processing or packaging
Light or lite	$\frac{1}{3}$ less calories or 50 percent less of a nutrient such as fat, sodium or sugar than the regular or reference food
Reduced	25 percent less calories, fat, saturated fat, cholesterol, sodium or sugar than the regular or reference food; words such as "lower" and "fewer" might also be used.
Lean	10 or fewer grams of fat, 4.5 or fewer grams of saturated fat and 95 or fewer milligrams of cholesterol per serving

Extra lean	5 or fewer grams of fat, 2 or fewer grams of saturated fat and 95 or fewer milligrams of cholesterol per serving
High	20 percent or more of the Percent Daily Value for a nutrient such as a vitamin, mineral, or fiber; "excellent source of" and "rich in" may also be used.
Good source	10 to 19 percent of the Percent Daily Value for a nutrient
More	10 percent or more of the Percent Daily Value for a nutrient; "enriched," "fortified" and "added" can also be used.
Healthy	Low in fat and saturated fat, 480 or fewer milligrams of sodium and at least 10 percent of the Percent Daily Value of vitamin A, vitamin C, calcium, iron, protein and fiber per serving

Notes

1. "Reference Daily Intake" (RDI) is a new term that replaces "U.S. Recommended Daily Allowance" (RDA). The percentages that a food contributes to the RDI for these nutrients are listed on the food label.
2. One teaspoon of table salt is approximately 6,000 milligrams; however, table salt is made up of 40 percent sodium and 60 percent chloride.

UNDERSTANDING PORTION CONTROL

Portion control may be one of the biggest factors causing the rising rate of obesity in this country. When it comes to food these days, bigger is better! There are "Super Meal Deals," "Super Size" and "50% More," and in many restaurants one meal is sometimes big enough to feed a family. Even too much of the right foods can make you gain weight. Learning appropriate portion sizes for different foods may be one of the most important skills you can learn when it comes to achieving and maintaining your healthy weight. It's a skill that takes time and practice to develop.

MASTERING PORTION CONTROL

- **Use the right tools.** Make sure you use measuring cups and spoons and a food scale to help you learn about the portion sizes you eat. These tools allow you to compare what you *really* eat with what you *should* eat. Measure all the foods you eat to learn about common servings.
- **Try eating with smaller plates and bowls.** This will help you avoid serving portions that are too large. It also makes smaller portions look bigger.

- **Cut foods, such as meat, into smaller pieces.** This also gives the appearance of more food and can help the meal last longer.
- **Buy meats and cheese that are already cut in appropriate serving sizes.**
- **Get out of the habit of eating everything on your plate, especially at restaurants.** Learn to stop eating before you're full; it's okay to leave some food behind. It's also okay to split a meal with a companion.

CONTROLLING MEAT, POULTRY AND FISH PORTIONS

One of the areas in which calories can easily add up unnoticed is the meat group. The recommended serving size for meat is three ounces. Unfortunately, we've gotten used to eating two to three times this amount. This is especially challenging when eating in restaurants. The average portion of meat served when dining out is 6 to 10 ounces. Remember, too, that restaurants don't always offer the leanest cuts of meat. With all of this in mind, it is a good idea to learn how to estimate a 3-ounce portion of meat:

- **Dinner-plate rule**: Imagine a standard dinner plate divided in quarters. Your meat serving should only fill one quarter of your plate. This means the other three-quarters should consist of complex carbohydrates—one-fourth starch and one-half vegetables/fruit.
- **Deck of cards rule**: An old favorite when trying to estimate 3-ounce portions of meat. A 3-ounce portion of meat should be no thicker and no wider than a standard deck of cards (or about the size of an audiocassette).
- **Lady's palm rule**: Three ounces of meat should fit nicely in the palm of an average-sized lady's hand.
- **Checkbook rule**: Three ounces of grilled fish is the size of a checkbook.
- **Eyeball rule**: This is another common rule. This is a simple rule of thumb that is easy to apply—if it looks too big, it probably is!

3 OUNCES OF MEAT, POULTRY OR FISH = $\frac{1}{4}$ OF THE PLATE

COMPLEX CARBOHYDRATES STARCH= $\frac{1}{4}$ OF THE PLATE

COMPLEX CARBOHYDRATES VEGETABLES & FRUIT= $\frac{1}{2}$ OF THE PLATE

When grocery shopping, keep in mind that chicken breasts are typically closer to 5 or 6 ounces each. Individual filet mignons, although they look small, are at least 6- to 8-ounce portions. It's a good idea to plan on cutting these portions in half before preparing. Eating a couple of ounces more than you should can add at least 100 calories!

SHORTCUTS FOR ESTIMATING PORTION SIZES

The key to moderation is controlling portion size. To achieve and maintain healthy body weight, learn to put into practice the concepts of "serving size." Use measuring cups, spoons and scales until you know appropriate portion sizes by heart. Here are some practical examples from the American Dietetics Association to help you estimate portion sizes when these tools aren't available:

- A medium potato should be the size of a computer mouse.
- An average bagel should be the size of a hockey puck.
- A cup of fruit is the size of a baseball.
- A cup of lettuce is four leaves.
- One ounce of cheese is the size of four dice.
- One ounce of snack foods, such as pretzels, is one handful.

SWEETNESS BY ANY OTHER NAME

Many different sugars are found naturally in foods. Sugars are also added in the preparation and manufacturing of many foods. In addition to tasting good, sugar plays several important roles in food. It gives certain foods their characteristic texture, color and consistency. You may have discovered the difference sugar makes when you reduce or substitute it in recipes.

Myths and misinformation about sugar and other sweeteners are very common. Common table sugar, or refined sugar, tops the misinformation list. You've probably also heard stories about saccharin and aspartame. Whether the sugar comes from the sugar bowl, honey, fruit, vegetables or milk, there's little difference from your body's viewpoint. In the end, your body converts sugars and starches from fruits, vegetables, grains and other foods to glucose. Along with fatty acids (fat), glucose is the main energy source for your body.

THE TRUTH ABOUT SUGAR

A gram of sugar contains four calories. That's less than half of the nine calories supplied by a gram of fat. A teaspoon of sugar contains 16 calories. A soft drink can have 9 to 12 teaspoons of sugar! What's the real problem? The estimated 150 pounds of sugar that the average American consumes each year adds up to a lot of calories. The bottom line is that too many calories are fattening, and it doesn't really matter whether the extra calories come from sugars, fat or protein. We gain weight when we take in more calories from our food than we expend in physical activity. The problem with sugar is that it often supplies empty calories (i.e., calories without the nutrition). Sugar is also often found in foods that are high in calories and fat. Because most of us have a sweet tooth, sugary foods often replace other more nutritious foods in our diets.

What's in a Name?

Acesulfame K	Glucose	Maple syrup
Aspartame	High-fructose corn syrup	Molasses
Brown sugar	Honey	Saccharin
Corn sweeteners	Lactose	Sorbitol
Dextrose	Maltose	Sugar
Fruit-juice concentrate	Mannitol	Xylitol

While there are some minor differences, your body treats these sugars much the same. In terms of nutritional value there's virtually no difference. The nonnutritive sweeteners—acesulfame K, aspartame and saccharin—add sweetness without the calories.

How Sweet It Is!

Nonnutritive sweeteners (also known as artificial, or intense, sweeteners) can give you the taste of sugar without the calories. It's important to read product labels; many foods labeled "sugar free" contain a sugar substitute, or nonnutritive sweetener. Even though foods made with nonnutritive sweeteners may be low in calories, many of them may also be low in nutrition. In a healthy eating plan, calories are not the only issue—you need to consider nutrition (i.e., vitamins, minerals, phytochemicals and fiber).

Four artificial sweeteners are commonly used today: aspartame, acesulfame potassium, saccharin and sucralose.

- **Aspartame** (e.g., NutraSweet and Equal) is a newer nonnutritive sweetener that actually contains calories. Because it's 180 times as sweet as sugar, you need only a tiny amount to sweeten food. It's actually a combination of two amino acids. One problem with aspartame is that it loses its sweetness when heated.

Consequently, you cannot use it in baked goods, such as cakes. You can use it in top-of-the-stove foods like pudding by adding it at the very end of cooking. Available scientific evidence does not support various health concerns reported by some individuals.

- **Acesulfame potassium** (e.g., Sunett) is 200 times sweeter than sugar and was first approved in 1988 as a tabletop sweetener. It is now approved for products such as baked goods, frozen desserts, candies and beverages. More than 90 studies verify its safety. It is often combined with other sweeteners. Worldwide, the sweetener is used in more than 4,000 products, according to its manufacturer, Nutrinova. It has excellent shelf life and does not break down when cooked or baked.

- **Saccharin** (e.g., Sweet'n Low) has been around for over 100 years. It's over 300 times sweeter than table sugar—a little goes a long way! Saccharin can be used in both hot and cold foods to make them sweeter. Substituting saccharin for sugar in baked goods may change their taste, texture and appearance. The risk of cancer associated with the use of saccharin in laboratory animals appears to be very low or nonexistent in humans.

- **Sucralose** (e.g., Splenda) is 600 times sweeter than sugar. It was approved in 1998 as a tabletop sweetener and for use in products such as baked goods, beverages, gum, frozen dairy desserts, fruit juices and gelatins. It is now approved as a general-purpose sweetener for all foods. It is bulked up with maltodextrin, a starchy powder, so it will measure more like sugar. It has a good shelf life and doesn't degrade when exposed to heat.

The key with both sugars and nonnutritive sweeteners is moderation. Let your overall goals of achieving and maintaining a healthy weight and good health help you decide what is best for you.

THE WISE USE OF SUGAR

Moderation, balance and variety are the keys to achieving and maintaining a healthy weight and good nutrition. Some dietitians actually advise people trying to lose weight to include some sugary foods in their diets. Eating plans that restrict certain foods are often too hard to maintain. Trying to eliminate certain foods often leads to an eventual slipup (i.e., you break down and eat that food). Slipups often lead to feelings of guilt and failure. The feelings cause many people to abandon their weight-loss efforts. Others report that there are certain foods they need to avoid in order to achieve their goals. If eating some sugary foods allows you to better reach your goals, that's okay. If eliminating sugary foods or using nonnutritive sweeteners helps you reach your goals, that's okay too! Many members of First Place have found success with this last approach. You decide what's best for you and your body.

There are no good or bad foods, only bad diets. Your eating plan should not focus on what you're eliminating but what you're adding—good nutrition, improved health and a higher quality of life.

CONVENIENCE FOODS—MAKING THE MOST OF YOUR TIME

Does life have you on the go? *Of course it does!* Our fast-paced lives require us to cook and eat on the run. Fortunately, grocery store aisles are filled with convenience foods of all types—frozen dinners, canned soups, ready-to-eat cereals— and they come in all types of packages—jars, cans, bottles, boxes and bags. These foods save time in our busy lives, but they can also be high in calories, fat, cholesterol, added sugars and sodium.

Don't let busyness become a roadblock to achieving and maintaining a healthy weight and following a nutritious eating plan. The keys to healthy nutrition are balance, moderation and variety, even in convenience foods.

READING LABELS

The most popular trend in convenience foods over the last several years is the introduction of *low-fat* foods. Low-fat versions of our favorite foods are everywhere. Recently one shopper was quoted as saying, "There's low fat, no fat, fat free, nonfat and 95 percent fat free—I spent half the morning at the grocery store just looking at brownie labels!" You may feel the same way. You would think with all the low-fat foods available, Americans would be losing pounds by the truckload. However, surveys show that Americans are gaining more weight than ever. There's one important thing to keep in mind: *Low fat doesn't necessarily mean low calorie!*

Product	Calories	Product	Calories
Chocolate cream-filled cookie	53	Fat-free version	55
Fig bar	60	Fat-free version	70
Granola cereal	130	Reduced-fat version	110
Breakfast bar	120	Reduced-fat version	120
3-ounce bagel	150	Today's bigger version	400

Next time you shop, compare the calories on the low-fat foods you buy with the regular versions. Is there really a difference? Compare serving sizes too. Sometimes the difference in calories is actually due to the smaller size!

CHOOSING HEALTHY CONVENIENCE FOODS

Dinners and single-item foods can fit into your daily balance of calories, fat, cholesterol, sodium, fiber and sugar. Use the following healthful guidelines to help you choose healthier convenience foods.

Look for Foods	Look for Clues on the Food Label	Know Your Daily Goal
Low in fat	3 or fewer grams of fat per serving	30 percent or less of total calories
Low in saturated fat	1 gram or less of saturated fat per serving	10 percent or less of total calories
Low in cholesterol	60 or fewer milligrams of cholesterol per serving	300 or fewer milligrams
Low in sodium	400 or fewer milligrams of sodium per serving	2,400 or fewer milligrams
High in fiber	2.5 or more grams of fiber per serving	25 to 30 grams of fiber
High in nutrients	10 percent or more of the RDI for one or more of the following: vitamin A, vitamin C, iron, calcium, protein and fiber	100 percent of the RDI

When choosing frozen dinners or entrees, use the following guidelines:

- Choose dinners that have fewer than 400 calories, 15 grams of fat, 5 grams of saturated fat and 800 milligrams of sodium.
- Choose entrees with fewer than 300 calories, 10 grams of fat and 4 grams of saturated fat.

USING CONVENIENCE FOODS

- Compare food labels when shopping for convenience foods. Choose the food with the lowest saturated fat, cholesterol and sodium.
- When cooking packaged foods such as instant noodles or macaroni and cheese, lower the fat and calories by using less butter or margarine than the directions call for. Use half of the seasoning packet, or use your own seasonings, to lower the sodium content. Add your own fresh or frozen vegetables to add fiber, vitamins and minerals.
- When buying canned meat such as chicken, tuna or salmon, choose water-packed varieties instead of oil-packed.
- Choose breakfast cereals with terms such as "high fiber," "whole grain" or "bran" on the label. Cereals that are high in fiber (>2.5 grams per serving) and low in added sugar are good choices.

- Canned or frozen fruits and vegetables are good choices, but watch out for sodium and added fats. Rinse vegetables, beans and canned meats with water to reduce the sodium content. Avoid canned and frozen vegetables with high-fat sauces.
- Limit use of frozen dinners and entrees with breaded or fried meats and vegetables.
- Buy prepackaged salads instead of individual ingredients. Buy products that contain an assortment of lettuce and other fresh vegetables. Be wary of salads that come with their own dressings and croutons, which are high in fat.
- Increase nutrients by balancing out your meal with a piece of fruit and a low-fat dairy product such as nonfat milk.
- Prepare your own healthy convenience foods by cooking your own recipes and freezing the leftovers in individual servings. Freezer bags and a variety of plastic containers make it convenient for you to store and reheat your meals.

CHANGING RECIPES

Low-fat cookbooks fill bookstore and library shelves. Perhaps you even have a collection of favorite cookbooks. If you like to cook and learn new recipes, that's great. But for most of us, learning all new recipes is not realistic. You don't have to buy a new cookbook or learn all new recipes to eat healthy and lose weight. You can make almost any recipe healthier with a few simple changes. Use the following tips to help turn your recipes into healthier alternatives.

JUST FOR STARTERS

- Which ingredients can be changed? Start by looking at ways to cut calories, fat, sugar and sodium.
- Find ways to increase nutrition by adding or substituting more healthful foods, such as whole grains, vegetables, legumes and fruits for less healthful foods, such as high-fat meats and refined grains.
- Make changes gradually to learn what works best. Changing ingredients can affect taste, texture and appearance.
- For that special occasion, don't change your favorite recipe—serve smaller portions.

CUT THE FAT

- Instead of frying meat, poultry and fish, broil, grill, roast or bake them. Use a rack or pans designed to catch drippings so that meat won't cook in its own fat. Use lean meats trimmed of visible fat and skin.
- Use vegetable-oil spray and nonstick pots and pans instead of oils and butter for cooking. Baste, broil and stir-fry using small amounts of oil, broth, water or fruit juice.

- Limit meat portions in your recipes to three ounces or less per serving. Make up for the reduced meat by adding more grains, rice or pasta, vegetables or legumes.
- Use meat alternatives—beans, lentils, peas and soy products—in recipes calling for meat.
- Drain fat from meat during or after cooking. Rinse cooked ground meat with hot water to remove much of the fat.
- Refrigerate soups and stews before serving. Remove the layer of fat that hardens after cooling.
- In recipes calling for eggs, use cholesterol-free egg substitutes or substitute two egg whites for every whole egg.
- To cut the fat called for in a recipe by $\frac{1}{3}$ to $\frac{1}{2}$, use vegetable oils instead of butter or shortening, and use low-fat dairy products.
- In recipes calling for cheese, use $\frac{1}{3}$ to $\frac{1}{2}$ of what the recipe calls for. Use low-fat cheese with 3 to 5 grams of fat per 1-ounce serving.
- Use nonfat sour cream or make your own by mixing $\frac{1}{2}$ cup of low-fat yogurt and $\frac{1}{2}$ cup of low-fat cottage cheese.
- Flavor with lemon juice and your favorite herbs and spices.
- Replace some of the fat in baked goods with fruit purées, such as prune, applesauce or banana, or nonfat dairy products such as nonfat yogurt. Use $\frac{1}{2}$ cup of puréed fruit in place of 1 cup of butter, shortening or oil. Don't get rid of all the fat. You may need to add 1 to 2 tablespoons of fat back into the recipe to achieve the best results.
- Use low-fat or nonfat cream cheese, sour cream, yogurt, mayonnaise and salad dressing instead of the full-fat versions.

CUT THE SUGAR

- Try using $\frac{1}{3}$ less sugar than what the recipe calls for.
- Substitute artificial sweeteners when appropriate. This will not work in many baked goods. Aspartame (e.g., NutraSweet, Equal) cannot be used in cooking—it loses its sweetness when heated. Sucralose (e.g., Splenda), however, can be used in cooking and baking.
- Learn to make special treats with fruits, such as fruit and yogurt smoothies, fruit pops, frozen bananas and trail mix.
- Experiment using fruit juice concentrates instead of sugar. You'll need to reduce the amount of overall liquid ingredients.
- Serve smaller portions of your favorite recipes.

CUT THE SODIUM

- Add flavor to vegetables, meats, poultry and fish with herbs and spices instead of using salt or high-sodium seasonings or sauces.
- Choose low-sodium versions of soups, broths and sauces.
- Eliminate or cut the salt in half for most of your recipes. Many seasoning packets in easy-to-fix meals (e.g., macaroni and cheese) are high in sodium. Use $\frac{1}{2}$ or less of the packet or substitute your own seasonings.
- Rinse canned vegetables with water to wash away extra sodium.

ADD FIBER, VITAMINS AND MINERALS

- Increase fiber by substituting whole-wheat flour, oats or cornmeal for some of the flour in recipes. Substitute ½ of white flour in a recipe with whole-wheat flour, or substitute ⅓ of white flour with oats.
- Add puréed fruits or vegetables in place of some of the water in recipes.
- Keep the peels on fruits and vegetables such as potatoes, carrots and apples.
- Add extra vegetables or grains such as rice, pasta or legumes to soups, sauces, salads and casseroles.
- Top a baked potato with steamed, fresh or stir-fried vegetables.

ADDING FLAVOR THE HEALTHY WAY

LOWERING SALT INTAKE

When it comes to health, sodium (salt) has drawn a considerable amount of attention because of its relationship to high blood pressure. High blood pressure is a leading risk factor for heart attack, stroke and kidney disease. Scientists have discovered that some people's blood pressure is very sensitive to excess sodium in the diet.

Because high blood pressure is such a serious health problem, the current U.S. Dietary Guidelines call for Americans to choose a diet moderate in salt and sodium. Most of the salt in the American diet comes from processed foods, however, not the salt shaker. Only about 15 percent of the sodium in the average diet is added in the kitchen or at the table. The top sources of salt in the diet include processed meats, prepackaged meals, fast foods, canned and dry soups, cheese, salted snack foods and certain condiments. The best way to learn how much sodium is in a food is to read the label. Foods that provide over 300 milligrams per serving are particularly high in sodium. For a single food item to carry the term "healthy" on the label, it must contain 360 or fewer milligrams of sodium per serving. Following is a list of foods particularly high in sodium:

- Canned and dry soups—1 cup contains 600-1,300 milligrams.
- Prepackaged meals (i.e., frozen dinners)—8 ounces contain 500-1,570 milligrams.
- Soy sauce—1 tablespoon contains 1030 milligrams.
- Salted popcorn—2½ cups contain 330 milligrams.
- Processed cheese and cheese spreads—1 ounce contains 340-450 milligrams.
- Cured ham—3 ounces contain 1,025 milligrams.

While we're born with a preference for sweet tastes, salt is an acquired taste. Many people find that after cutting down on salt, many foods that they used to enjoy taste too salty. Cut down gradually to give your taste buds time to adapt. To be sure you consume no more than 2,400 milligrams of sodium per day, try following some of these helpful tips:

- Choose foods that are naturally low in sodium, such as fresh fruits and vegetables.
- Break the habit of adding salt during cooking—there's no reason to salt cooking water—or at the table.
- Rinse canned meats, legumes and vegetables under cold water to remove excess salt.
- Eat a variety of foods during a single meal to stimulate the taste buds.
- Eat meals slowly and savor the flavor and aroma of each bite.
- In most recipes you can cut the salt in half (or more).
- For meals with dried seasoning packets, use half or less of the packet to cut down on the sodium.
- Learn to season foods with herbs, spices, fruit juice and flavored vinegars.
- Limit processed meats such as ham, bacon, hot dogs and luncheon meats.
- Limit high-salt condiments such as soy sauce, steak sauce, barbecue sauce, mustard and ketchup.
- Buy reduced-salt or low-salt snack foods.
- Limit consumption of olives, pickles, relishes and many salad dressings which are loaded with salt.
- When eating out ask for meals to be prepared with less salt, ask for sauces to be served on the side and avoid using the salt shaker.

HERBS AND SPICES

Adding herbs, spices or other flavorings is great way to make tasty dishes that are low in sodium. You'll have to experiment to find out what works best for you. Following are some tips on using and storing herbs and spices:

- Read the label; some premixed spices contain salt.
- Store herbs and spices in a cool, dark place and in tight containers. Avoid heat, moisture and light.
- Date dry herbs and spices when you buy them; shelf life is about one year.
- Test the freshness of herbs by rubbing them between your fingers and checking the aroma.
- Crumbling dry herbs between your fingers before using releases more flavor.
- Liquid brings out the flavor of dried herbs and spices.

- If you use fresh herbs, store them in a plastic bag in the refrigerator. Before using, wash and pat dry.
- For soups and stews—dishes that have to cook awhile—add herbs and spices toward the end of cooking.
- For chilled dishes or meats, the earlier you add the herbs and spices the better the flavor.
- When trying new herbs and spices, add them gradually to the dish—you can always add more.

SEASONING IDEAS FOR MEAT AND VEGETABLES

Beef	Bay leaf, dry mustard, marjoram, nutmeg, onion, pepper, sage, thyme
Fish	Curry powder, dill, dry mustard, lemon juice, marjoram, paprika, pepper
Poultry	Ginger, marjoram, oregano, paprika, rosemary, sage, tarragon, sage, thyme
Carrots	Cinnamon, cloves, marjoram, nutmeg, rosemary, sage
Corn	Cumin, curry powder, green pepper, onion, paprika, parsley
Green Beans	Dill, curry powder, lemon juice, marjoram, oregano, tarragon, thyme
Peas	Basil, dill, ginger, marjoram, onion, parsley, sage
Potatoes	Basil, dill, garlic, onion, paprika, parsley, rosemary, sage
Squash	Allspice, basil, cinnamon, curry powder, ginger, marjoram, nutmeg, onion, rosemary, sage
Tomatoes	Basil, bay leaf, dill, marjoram, onion, oregano, parsley, pepper, thyme

MEATLESS MEALS

For many people, meat is part of their daily meal plan. Unfortunately, meat is at the top of the list of foods that contribute the most calories, fat, saturated fat and cholesterol to the American diet. You don't have to eat meat every day to meet your body's nutritional needs. Research shows that an eating plan high in fruits, vegetables, whole grains and low-fat dairy products reduces the risk for many diseases, such as coronary heart disease, high blood pressure, diabetes and some forms of cancer. While we're not recommending you eat only vegetables and water, eating a few meatless meals may be a healthy addition to your eating plan.

REDUCING MEAT CONSUMPTION

Following the First Place Live-It plan will give your body the protein it needs. However, most Americans eat much more protein than they need for good health. Keep in mind what counts as a serving (see page 159). Consider the typical portion sizes served in most restaurants and what you eat at home. As you'll probably realize, it's easy to eat more meat than you need.

One smart way to reduce your meat intake—and the fat and cholesterol that come with it—is to choose small portions of lean meats. Another way is to substitute other good sources of protein for meals that usually contain meat. Plant proteins can meet your body's daily needs, as long as you choose from a wide variety of protein-rich plant foods, such as whole grains, legumes, vegetables, low-fat dairy products, seeds and nuts. Remember, however, that some meatless sources of protein, such as cheese, nuts and seeds, can be high in calories and fat.

Caution: Besides meat, what other food provides the most calories, fat, saturated fat and cholesterol in the American diet? Cheese! It's common for people who are trying to eat less meat to substitute cheese instead. Watch out! Ounce for ounce, regular cheese has more fat and saturated fat than many cuts of meat and can be higher in cholesterol as well. Be sure to choose reduced-fat cheeses as often as possible.[1] Choose cheeses with 3 to 5 grams of fat per ounce, and remember a good rule of thumb is: "The whiter the cheese, the lower the fat."

The legume family—beans, peas, lentils and soybeans—provides a good source of protein. Legumes are also good sources of carbohydrates, B vitamins and many other essential vitamins and minerals. They're a great source of soluble fiber, which helps lower blood cholesterol levels. Soy products, such as tofu, are especially good substitutes for animal proteins. Use legumes as the main part of any meal or add them to dishes such as soups, sauces and casseroles that typically call for meat. Choose any variety you like—kidney beans, navy beans, black beans, peas and lentils—and in any form—dried, canned, fresh or frozen.

CHOOSING ALTERNATIVES

To help get you started, here are some suggestions for meatless meals:
- Vegetarian pizza: Instead of meats, pile on the vegetables.
- Spaghetti with meatless sauce: Add beans or other vegetables to the sauce instead of meat.
- Casseroles: Use beans, whole grains or extra vegetables for some or all of the meat in the recipe.

- Bean burrito: Avoid beans refried in lard, and go easy on the cheese.
- Vegetarian soups: Replace the meat in soups with beans or whole grains, such as rice or pasta.
- Salads: Use beans, such as kidney or garbanzo, or low-fat cottage cheese instead of meat toppings.

DINING IN OR OUT

Try some of these helpful ideas for meatless meals, or come up with your own.

Breakfast

- Select whole-grain, ready-to-eat cereal and nonfat milk.
- Choose whole-grain toast, English muffin, bagel or toaster waffle with jam or jelly. Add nonfat cream cheese or a little peanut butter as a source of protein.
- Low-fat yogurt is a great source of protein, calcium and other nutrients.

Lunch or Dinner

- Eat fresh vegetable salad, but go easy on the cheese. Add beans, peas, other legumes, nuts and seeds to boost protein, vitamins and minerals.
- Choose broth-based instead of cream-based meatless soups. Rice, pasta and other grains such as barley or tabouli are good substitutes for meat in many soups.
- Vegetable sandwiches are a good choice, but watch out for cheese and high-fat spreads such as cream cheese or mayonnaise. Try a vegetarian burger for a change of pace. These are usually made with whole grains, soy protein and other vegetables. They're lower in calories, fat and cholesterol than the traditional burger. Experiment until you find one you like.
- Prepare stir-fry with legumes, tofu or extra vegetables instead of meat.

Other Tips for Meatless Meals

- Choose restaurants with vegetarian choices; many ethnic cuisines offer meatless dishes.
- Order salads, soups, breads and fruits if a restaurant doesn't offer meatless dishes.
- When traveling, call the airline at least 48 hours in advance to request a meatless meal.

Note

1. Cheeses labeled "low sodium" will be higher in fat than cheeses with higher sodium content.

OFF TO A GOOD START

Breakfast may be the most important meal of the day. After all, your body hasn't had any food for 8 to 12 hours—it's time to break the fast. After a night's sleep, your body needs a fresh supply of fuel and nutrients to start the day. Your mind needs energy to be sharp. Your muscles need energy to keep you on the move. A healthy breakfast gives your body what it needs.

RESEARCH RESULTS

- Several studies show that breakfast eaters perform better mentally and physically.
- Some studies suggest that breakfast skippers are more likely to overeat later in the day. Approaching snack time or lunch on an empty stomach can lead to poor choices and overeating.
- Studies show that regular breakfast eaters consume more nutrients throughout the day. Regular breakfast eaters are more likely to get adequate levels of minerals, such as calcium, phosphorus and magnesium and vitamins, such as riboflavin, folate and vitamins A, C, and B_{12}.
- One study of nearly 3,500 men and women found that regular cereal eaters eat less fat during the day, have a lower cholesterol intake and eat more fiber. They also have lower blood cholesterol levels. All these factors add up to a lower risk for heart disease.

Unfortunately, despite all the benefits of starting the day with a healthy breakfast, it's the meal most often skipped.

HEALTHY CHOICES

While eating any kind of breakfast may be better than skipping, it's important to make healthy choices. Soft drinks, sugary cereals, pastries, fried potatoes and high-fat meats are not a healthy way to go. These foods supply calories your body needs for energy but can be high in fat, cholesterol and sugar and low in vitamins, minerals and fiber. A balanced breakfast will give you the sustained energy and nutrients your body needs.

Try to eat a well-balanced breakfast high in complex carbohydrates, some protein and a little fat. Whole-grain cereals and breads, nonfat milk, yogurt, fruit and even eggs are good choices. These foods stay with you longer and give you the energy you need to make it through the morning. Many breakfast foods are high in simple sugars and can quickly leave you feeling hungry again.

CEREAL

Hot and cold cereals are a great start to any day. Fortified cereals provide vitamins, such as folate and other B vitamins, and minerals, such as iron and calcium. Adding low-fat milk boosts the protein, B vitamins and minerals such as calcium, phosphorus and magnesium. High-fiber cereals help keep your digestive system working regularly and provide other important health benefits. Balance out your breakfast and get a start on your five-a-day goal by eating fresh fruit with your cereal.

Read the Nutrition Facts label and the ingredient list to find the cereals best for you. Look for high-fiber, low-sugar and vitamin-fortified brands. You want the first ingredients listed to be whole grains or rolled oats. Look for cereals with 5 to 10 grams of sugar or fewer and more than 2.5 grams of fiber per serving. Low-fat cereals have no more than 2 to 3 grams of fat. And watch out for granola, which is often high in fat and sugar. Some varieties of cereal are fortified with 100 percent of the Recommended Daily Intake for vitamins and minerals—just make sure to finish the milk in the bottom of the bowl!

CREATIVE SOLUTIONS

What are some creative and enjoyable ways you can begin to make a healthy breakfast part of your daily routine? Try these tips to help get you started:

- Make sure you wake up in time to fit in a good breakfast—10 to 15 minutes is all you need. To save time, prepare for breakfast before you go to bed.
- If you don't have time to eat at home or if you're not hungry first thing in the morning, drink a small glass of low-fat milk, or fruit or vegetable juice on the way to work. You can pack a bagel, breakfast bar, yogurt, peanut-butter sandwich, cheese and crackers or fresh fruit to eat on the way to or at work.
- Make eating breakfast a family affair. Start the day connecting with your family and fueling your bodies for the day ahead. What a great time to start the day with prayer!
- It takes just minutes to make a delicious smoothie. Simply mix nonfat yogurt, frozen fruit and juice or milk in a blender—experiment! Drink it while you're getting ready or on your way to work.
- Pop frozen waffles (preferably whole grain) into the toaster and top with jam, jelly, yogurt, low-fat cream cheese or peanut butter. You can do the same with whole-grain breads, bagels or English muffins.
- Skip the fat-laden breakfast sandwiches offered by fast-food chains. Make your own from low-fat cheese, lean ham or turkey, bread, bagel or an English muffin.

- Who says you have to eat a traditional breakfast in the morning? Leftover vegetable pizza, grilled-cheese sandwiches, burritos and other lunch and dinnertime favorites are options you can choose. You can have a quick and nutritious breakfast by reheating leftovers.

BREAKFAST IN THE FAST LANE

Do you find yourself eating breakfast away from home or in the car? The following will help you make healthy choices:

- Hot and cold cereals are a good choice at any restaurant.
- Pancakes and waffles can be a good choice if you go easy on the butter or margarine. Top them with fresh fruit, jam, jelly or syrup.
- Order fruit juice and low-fat milk instead of coffee or a soft drink for breakfast.
- Eggs are a good choice because they are a good source of protein, iron and vitamin A. It's the egg yolks that are high in cholesterol; ask for scrambled eggs without the yolk or made with an egg substitute.
- A bagel or English muffin is a good choice, but watch the butter and cream cheese. Most muffins are high in fat and calories, as are pastries, croissants and biscuits.

TAKE TIME FOR A HEALTHY LUNCH

Do you take time for lunch? Our busy lifestyles often lead to lunch on the run. For many, lunch is a popular social time rather than a time to nourish the body. Some of us are so busy we don't even take time for lunch.

The most popular lunchtime fares are sandwiches, hamburgers and salads. The truth of the matter is that traditional sandwiches and salads may not be any lower in fat and calories than the fast-food burger!

Avoiding lunch leads to fatigue, hunger and overeating later in the day or night. Extreme hunger can also lead to cravings for junk food and binge eating. On the positive side, a nutritious lunch can give your body the fuel it needs to meet the physical and mental demands of the rest of the day. Lunchtime can also offer a much-needed break after a hard morning of work. A light nutritious meal plus 10 to 20 minutes of moderate activity during the lunch hour is a great way to achieve good health and a healthy weight. Eating too much fat, calories and sugar may do you in for the rest of the day.

EXCUSES FOR NOT EATING A HEALTHY LUNCH

- No time! Even if you can't stop for a relaxing lunch break, you can take a few minutes to eat some nutritious foods. It's easy to eat a sandwich, cheese and crackers, yogurt or fresh fruit—if you have prepared ahead of time.
- I don't need the calories! This is *not* a good reason to skip lunch. Your body needs energy and nutrients throughout the day. Skipping meals only leads to overeating later in the day. With every meal you skip, you rob your body of important nutrients and sources for the energy needed to make it through the afternoon hours.

Examine your reasons for not eating a healthy lunch. What are some possible solutions? What are the benefits of eating a nutritious lunch? Begin making plans to make a nutritious lunch a regular part of your day.

EATING OUT

Eating a healthy lunch is now easier than ever. Fast-food and other restaurants now offer several nutritious and low-fat options. Of course, most menus offer selections that are high in calories, fat and cholesterol, and low in fresh fruits, vegetables and whole grains. The key is to plan ahead and order what you know is best.

Best Bets for a Healthy Lunch

- A fresh salad with an assortment of colorful vegetables, low-fat dressing (*On the side please!*), grilled chicken, grilled chicken sandwich (*Hold the mayo!*), bean and cheese burrito (*Go easy on the cheese and add extra lettuce and tomato!*), small hamburger or baked potato (*Toppings on the side!*) are all good choices. All these meals have fewer than 400 calories and 30 percent or less fat.
- Deli sandwiches can be a healthy choice. Choose lean meats such as turkey, ham or roast beef. Ask for mustard or light mayonnaise. Ask for less meat (usually half the typical serving), more lettuce, tomato and other vegetables, and whole-grain bread. Hold the chips or fries.
- Pizza can be a good choice if you choose carefully. Stick to vegetable pizza and ask for less cheese and more sauce and vegetables. Limit yourself to one or two slices of thin-crust pizza. Eat a salad too (low-fat dressing on the side).
- Pick out three or four restaurants where you know you can get healthy foods. Suggest to friends and colleagues that you eat at these places when you eat out for lunch.

Worst Bets for a Healthy Lunch

- A hamburger and fries, a tuna-salad sandwich or a chicken Caesar salad can supply half of the fat and calories recommended for an entire day. The typical deli-style sandwich piled with meat, mayonnaise and cheese—and bacon if it's a club sandwich—is not any better.
- Is salad a healthy choice? A ladle of regular salad dressing contains four tablespoons—nearly 300 calories of fat or half of your recommended daily intake.
- Fried foods—french fries, fried chicken and fish, burgers, tacos, etc.—should not be a regular part of the lunchtime meal. Frying can double the fat and calories.
- Portion sizes can be two to three times what you need—split a meal with a companion or take some home to eat for another meal.

PACKING YOUR LUNCH

Packing a healthy lunch starts with planning. A healthy brown-bag lunch starts in the grocery store. Plan ahead to buy a variety of nutritious foods that you enjoy and are convenient for you to prepare and pack along. When preparing your lunch, remember the key principles of variety, balance and moderation.

- You'll need an assortment of plastic containers, plastic bags and maybe even a thermos. An insulated lunch bag or cooler can keep foods cool if you don't have access to a refrigerator.
- Canned and frozen fruits, vegetables and beans can be placed in individual-sized plastic containers. You can do the same with soups. Add your own seasonings when packing. Your meal is now ready to heat in a microwave when you're ready.
- Take along low-fat dairy foods. Milk can be kept cool in a thermos and yogurt can stay at room temperature for several hours. Mix canned fruit or fresh vegetables with cottage cheese in a plastic container.
- Keep plenty of your favorite fruits and vegetables on hand wherever you are. If they need cutting or peeling, do it the night before. Better yet, prepare them as soon as you come home from the grocery store. Store them away in plastic bags or containers so they're ready to go when you are.
- Make a sandwich with lean meat and fresh vegetables the night before. Place it in a sandwich container or plastic bag and it will be ready to go when you leave in the morning.
- Make lunch quick and easy by bringing leftovers. Most leftovers can be easily reheated in a microwave. When cooking at home, make extra portions and store the extras individually for a ready-to-serve lunch.

- Packing your own lunch also saves money; it's much cheaper to pack your own than to eat out. The savings over an entire year could pay for a health club membership or home exercise equipment!
- Always have enjoyable standbys when you find yourself short on time or choices. Dried and canned soups and fruits, crackers, peanut butter, oatmeal, cereal, bagels and energy bars can be kept on hand in a pantry or desk drawer for a quick and easy lunch anytime.

OUTSMARTING THE SNACK ATTACK!

If you want to lose weight, you've got to cut out the snacks!

Have you heard that before? Actually, it's not the snacking that's bad, it's the usual snack choices—chips, crackers, dips, cookies, candy bars, etc.—that are the problem. The truth is that your body works best when it refuels every four to six hours. The best way to fuel your body is to eat light, well-balanced meals and two or three healthy snacks. Snacking may even help you lose weight by taming your appetite, thus preventing the tendency to overeat and make poor choices. Learn to make healthy snacks a part of your daily eating plan.

SNACK FACTS

Surveys suggest that 99 percent of Americans snack, and 75 percent do so one or more times each day. How much do we spend on snacking? Over $40 million each day. Snacking accounts for nearly 25 percent of daily calories, and by the end of one year the average person has consumed over 22 pounds of snack foods, mostly chips, pretzels, puffs and candy. On the positive side, many of our favorite snack foods now come in low-fat versions. On the down side, many of these are still high in calories and low in nutrition.

Why do you snack?

☐ To satisfy hunger   ☐ To relax

☐ To satisfy cravings   ☐ For enjoyment and pleasure

☐ To boost energy   ☐ For nourishment

☐ To fight bordeom and pass time   ☐ Other_____

It's important to understand the reasons why you snack. It's also important to know how your typical snack foods stack up nutritionally. Use snacks to satisfy hunger, nourish your body, boost your energy and help you reach your goals for a healthy weight.

HEALTHY SNACKING

The key to healthy nutrition is variety, balance and moderation. With these principles in mind, snacking can be an important part of a healthy eating plan. Snack time can be a great way to get in your daily servings of fruits, vegetables and whole grains. Low-fat dairy foods such as milk and yogurt also make a healthy snack. Keep a supply of healthy snacks in convenient locations. Concentrate on complex carbohydrates and low-fat proteins. Do whatever you can to avoid those high-fat, high-sugar treats that always seem to show up at home, work and social occasions. Healthy beverages can also be great at snack time; water, fruit or vegetable juice, and low-fat milk are your best choices.

The important thing to remember about snacking is that when you eat is not as important as what and how much you eat. When it comes to weight control the issue is total calories—not when or how often you eat. As for snacking, eat only when you're hungry and stop when you're full!

HOW SNACKS STACK UP

Snack	Calories	Fat (grams)
Ice cream (1 cup)	~ 300	~ 15
Candy bar (2 ounces)	~ 250	~ 12
Mixed nuts (1 ounce or 20 nuts)	~ 200	~ 15
Fried chips (1 ounce or 10 chips)	~ 160	~ 10
Microwave popcorn (3 cups)	~ 150	~ 10
Nonfat fruit yogurt (1 cup)	~ 120	0
Baked chips (1 ounce or 13 chips)	~ 110	~ 1
Pretzels (1 ounce or 9 pretzels)	~ 110	~ 1
Fresh fruit (1 medium)	~ 60	trace
Air-popped popcorn (3 cups)	~ 50	trace
Vegetable (1/2 cup)	~ 25	trace

PLAN AHEAD

Stock your home, office and workout bag with a variety of healthy snacks so you'll always have something healthy on hand when hunger strikes. Buy several plastic containers, plastic bags, a thermos and an insulated lunch bag or cooler to make it easy for you to carry snacks with you. Keep a special shopping list to help you remember to stock up on healthy snack foods. Instead of looking for low-fat versions of your favorite processed snack foods, choose foods such as whole-grain breads and crackers, fruits, vegetables, rice cakes and low-fat yogurt.

PACKABLE SNACKS

animal cookies	fresh, canned, and	low-fat cheese	low-fat yogurt
bagels	dried fruits	low-fat cookies	nonfat chips
bread sticks	fruit juice (single servings)	low-fat granola bars	plain popcorn
cheese sticks	graham crackers	low-fat popcorn	pretzels
energy bars	instant oatmeal	low-fat peanut butter	ready-to-eat cereal
fig bars	lean luncheon and	low-fat whole-grain	water
	canned meats	crackers	

HEALTHY SNACK CHOICES

50-Calorie Snacks	Exchanges	50-Calorie Snacks	Exchanges
30 small pretzel sticks	1 bread	1 kiwi fruit	1 fruit
1 tangerine	½ fruit	3 apricots	1 fruit
2 tomatoes	2 fruits	½ cup blueberries	½ fruit
1 cup zucchini sticks	1 vegetable	10 ripe olives	1 fat
1 large dill pickle	½ vegetable	½ cup orange juice	1 fruit
1 (4-inch) rice cake	½ bread	1 medium cucumber	2 vegetables
1 cup tomato juice	1½ vegetables	4 slices melba toast	½ bread
1 carrot	1½ vegetables	1 medium peach	½ fruit
2 gingersnaps	½ bread, ½ fat	1 cup strawberries	½ fruit
¾ cup raspberries	1 fruit	6 cherry tomatoes	1 vegetable
12 strawberries	½ fruit	¾ cup consommé or broth	½ meat
½ cup fat-free milk	½ milk	12 whole radishes	½ vegetable
8 celery ribs	2 vegetables	1 caramel popcorn cake	1 bread
4 saltine crackers	½ bread, ½ fat	2 slices garlic crisp bread	½ bread
2 fortune cookies	1 bread (sugar)	½ cup mandarin orange slices	½ fruit
2 cups broccoli florets	2 vegetables	¼ cup tropical fruit salad	½ fruit

Eating Healthy on the Go

NUTRITION WHILE TRAVELING

Whether traveling for business or pleasure, eating healthy on the road can be difficult. The secret is *getting away* without *getting back* all the weight you've worked so hard *getting off*. With a little planning, you can keep on track when you travel.

HOW TO EAT HEALTHY

Part of the enjoyment of traveling is the chance to try out new cuisine. When you travel, allow yourself to enjoy new foods. A *few* choices that are higher in fat, sugar and calories are okay.

The key is to plan ahead how you want to eat while traveling and stick to it. Get support from your traveling companions. Let them know that you plan to eat healthy. It's much easier to make healthy choices when you have the support of others. Plus, you might be a positive influence on them!

On the Road

- **Pack your own snacks.** Good choices include bagels, fresh or dried fruits, raw vegetables, low-fat crackers, rice cakes, pretzels and cereal bars. By having your own snacks with you, you can avoid becoming too hungry and then overeating the first chance you get.
- **Eat a healthy meal before you hit the road.** Filling up before you leave will help you avoid making less healthful choices while on the road.
- **Pack a cooler.** Take along sandwiches, fruits, vegetables, low-fat yogurt and healthy beverages such as water, juice and low-fat milk.
- **When eating at fast-food restaurants, avoid fried foods and supersized or deluxe meals.** Choose regular-sized portions and choose grilled-chicken or other lean-meat sandwiches, baked potatoes (but easy on the cheese!) and fresh salads.
- **Stop regularly for a little physical activity,** such as stretching and a short walk—every little bit helps!

In the Air

- **Don't eat the airline meal just because it's offered.** Ask yourself if you're hungry. What are your meal plans when you arrive? If you're not hungry or you're planning to eat when you arrive, save the calories. Instead, ask for milk or juice and a snack to curb your appetite.
- **Call at least 48 hours in advance to request a special meal: low-fat, low-cholesterol or vegetarian.**
- **Water is a great way to stay hydrated in the pressurized environment.** Choose fruit or vegetable juice, low-fat milk or water instead of soft drinks or other beverages. Water is a great way to stay hydrated while you're in the air.
- **Bring your own food in a carry-on bag.** Good choices include fresh and dried fruit, ready-to-eat cereals, bagels, crackers and low-fat cheese.
- **Eat a healthy meal or snack before you arrive at the airport or board the airplane.**
- **Walk around the airport.** This is a good idea not only for the exercise, but it also gives you the opportunity to stake out healthy food options.
- **When the "fasten seat belt" sign goes off, get up and walk up and down the aisle every 20 minutes or so.**

Out on the Town

- **Choose restaurants wisely.** You can call the restaurant ahead of time to check out the menu. Ask if they prepare food to order or accept special requests.
- **Watch out for those large portions.** Try to choose smaller portions or share larger portions with a companion. Three ounces of meat is about the size of a deck of playing cards.
- **Don't skip meals to save up for that special meal.** Balance out a meal higher in fat and calories by making healthier choices during the day.
- **If you eat dessert, share it with a companion or take only a few bites.**
- **Beware of buffets.** Load up on fresh fruits, vegetables and other low-fat choices. Don't load up your plate just because it's "all you can eat." Rather than trying all the foods, pick one or two of your favorites and keep your portions small.
- **Eating smaller portions is a good way to enjoy a variety of foods.** Balance less healthy choices with better choices such as fresh fruits, vegetables and whole-grain foods.
- **When dining in foreign countries, you may need to avoid raw fruits and vegetables, raw or partly cooked meats and tap water.** A good rule to remember: If it's been boiled, cooked, bottled or peeled, it's probably okay.

More Helpful Tips

- **Stay at hotels and resorts that offer healthy dining options.**
- **Start each day with a healthy breakfast.** Fresh fruit; toast, a bagel or English muffin with jam; hot or cold cereal; and low-fat yogurt are good choices. Fresh-squeezed juice and low-fat or nonfat milk are good beverage choices. Limit your intake of eggs, sausage, bacon, sweet rolls, donuts, croissants and fried potatoes.
- **Carry snacks with you to business meetings or while sightseeing.** Try to avoid becoming overly hungry. If you wait too long between meals, you're more likely to overeat or make less healthy choices.
- **Make time for physical activity.**

WATCH FOR HIDDEN FATS

When eating away from home, it can be difficult to estimate how much fat is in a meal. It's important to estimate hidden fats in food because extra calories can add up quickly. Just one teaspoon of oil or one tablespoon of salad dressing has 5 grams of fat and 45 calories. Considering that a ladle of dressing at most salad bars is three or four tablespoons, it's easy to see how fat calories can add up!

ESTIMATING THE HIDDEN FATS

- Vegetables cooked with oil or butter—add ½ to 1 fat exchange
- Any fried food (meat, vegetable, French fries)—add 1 to 2 fat exchanges
- Tuna, chicken or potato salad—add 2 fat exchanges
- Salad with regular dressing—add 2 fat exchanges
- Gravy and special sauces—add 1 fat exchange

The best way to control hidden fats when eating out is to ask that foods be prepared without added fats and that salad dressing, gravies and sauces be served on the side.

LIFE IN THE FAST-FOOD LANE

Eating in the fast-food lane has become a way of life for many of us. Life has us on the go, so we have to eat on the go. Why do people choose to eat fast foods? *Taste*, *convenience* and *price* top the list. These reasons are important, but good nutrition and health should be at the top of your list.

FAST-FOOD FARE

What foods do you think of when you think fast food: burgers and fries, fried chicken, tacos and burritos, soft drinks? A fast-food meal can easily top 1,000 calories and give you a day's worth of fat, cholesterol and sodium. Believe it or not, you can also make healthy fast-food choices. Today, most fast-food restaurants offer a variety of foods such as grilled chicken, salads, baked potatoes and deli-style sandwiches. Of course, fresh fruits and vegetables are hard to find. The key is to plan ahead and be prepared to make healthy choices. Look for ways to trim fat, cut calories and add variety whenever you can. Always keep your goals of a healthy weight and good nutrition in mind. Here are some helpful tips—pick the ones that will work best for you.

Eating on the Go

- **Order individual items rather than the special meal deal.** One item that is higher in calories and fat may be okay, but add fries and a soft drink and you may double the calories and fat.
- **Watch out for words such as "deluxe," "supersize" or "jumbo."** Order the regular or small size instead. A single slice of cheese on a small burger adds calcium. Think nutrition—add the cheese and cut the fries.
- **Choose sandwiches with grilled chicken or fish, or lean roast beef, turkey or ham.** Ask for low-fat toppings such as mustard or low-fat salad dressing instead of mayonnaise or special sauce.
- **If you're having fast-food for one meal, choose healthier foods the rest of the day.** Don't forget your fruits and vegetables. You can even carry a piece of fruit with you to eat with your meal.

Lettuce Works

- **Beware—salads can have more calories, fat and sodium than a burger and fries!** Limit items such as cheese, croutons, bacon, eggs, nuts and creamy salad dressings. Add more vegetables instead.
- **Always order salad dressing on the side.** Use the low-fat dressing whenever possible. Salsa and low-fat cottage cheese are also good choices. Add flavor with fresh fruits, peppers and other vegetables.

- Limit special salads such as potato, macaroni, tuna and chicken. These salads are often made with mayonnaise or high-fat salad dressing. Choose coleslaw or bean salad made with vinaigrette instead.

Potato Toppings

- Plain baked potatoes are low in calories and fat and are a good source of fiber and vitamin C. Limit toppings such as butter, cheese, bacon and sour cream.
- Healthier choices include small amounts of margarine and low-fat sour cream. Other good toppings include low-fat cottage cheese, plain yogurt and salsa. Pack on the nutrition by adding lots of fresh vegetables.

Fast-Food Olé

- Choose grilled chicken (without the skin), beans or vegetables instead of beef or cheese on tostados, tacos or burritos. Ask for your bean burrito to be prepared with less cheese. Order soft tortillas rather than fried.
- Go easy on—or abstain from—cheese, sour cream and guacamole. Add more lettuce, tomatoes and salsa.

The Orient Express

- Asian take-out is one fast-food option that offers a variety of vegetables. Watch out, however, portion sizes can be large! Make a plan to split a dish with a companion or save some for another meal.
- Ask before you order. Many Asian dishes include fried meats. Order steamed rice instead of fried rice, forego the fried egg roll and ask for extra vegetables.

The Pizza Plan

- Choose thin crust over thick crust or deep dish.
- Avoid meats such as ground beef and pepperoni. These meats are higher in fat and sodium. Instead, ask for extra tomato sauce, fresh vegetables and less cheese.
- Limit yourself to one or two slices.
- Order a salad. A healthy salad will add variety and nutrition to your meal.

Drink Up

- Choose low-fat milk or natural fruit juice to drink. This will boost the nutrition of any fast-food meal. Water is always a good choice!

- Remember that some milk shakes can equal the calories and fat of an entire meal. Keep this in mind, and cut back in other areas if you order the shake.

A Healthy Beginning

- If breakfast is most often your fast-food meal, choose a plain bagel, toast or English muffin with jelly, jam or low-fat cream cheese. Skip the croissant and biscuits, which are high in fat and calories.
- Cold or hot cereals with nonfat milk, pancakes without butter or plain scrambled eggs are also good choices. Limit high-fat meats such as bacon and sausage and watch out for fried potatoes.

DINING OUT ASIAN STYLE

Asian restaurants have become an American favorite. With a variety of foods, cooking styles and atmospheres, they offer both enjoyable and healthful dining. Asian restaurants often use low-fat cooking methods and lean meats, fresh vegetables, rice and noodles. However, these same nutritious foods are often deep-fried or stir-fried and served with high-sodium sauces. Add in the typically large portions and an egg roll, and a single meal can easily top 1,500 calories.

WHAT TO ORDER

With the diversity of Asian cuisine—Chinese, Japanese, Thai, Korean and Vietnamese—and cooking styles, it's important to know how to read menus. The following chart of the most common menu items and terms will aid you in choosing wisely. Choose low-fat items more often and high-fat and high-sodium items less often.

Low in Fat	High in Fat	High in Sodium
Barbecued	Coconut milk	Black bean sauce
Bean curd	Duck	Hoisin sauce
Braised	Egg rolls	Miso sauce
Roasted or grilled	Fried or crispy	Most soups
Simmered	Fried rice or noodles	Oyster sauce
Steamed	Peanuts or cashews	Pickled
Stir-fried	Tempura	Soy sauce
Water chestnuts	Wonton	Teriyaki sauce

Did You Know?

🍎 **Some Asian sauces, such as sweet-and-sour and plum sauce, are actually low in fat, calories and sodium.** The problem is that dishes served with these sauces often consist of deep-fried meats.

🍎 **A tablespoon of soy sauce has nearly 1,000 milligrams of sodium**—almost half of the recommended daily intake of 2,400 milligrams.

🍎 **While Asian cuisine uses lots of vegetables, salads are somewhat unusual.** The exceptions are Thai and Vietnamese cuisine, which offer a variety of salads, including garden salads.

🍎 **The trendy Japanese sushi—a combination of raw fish, vinegared rice and often seaweed—is actually low in fat, calories and sodium, depending on the dipping sauce.**

HEALTHY CHOICES FOR ANY OCCASION

Appetizers and Soups

Traditional appetizers such as egg rolls, wonton and fried shrimp are high in calories and fat. Ask if the restaurant offers steamed spring rolls or steamed dumplings instead. If you choose the egg roll, eat only the inside.

Many Asian soups, such as hot-and-sour and egg-drop, offer a great way to start a meal. These broth-based soups are low in calories and fat.

The Main Meal

Asian dishes are usually served in large portions—enough for at least two people. Remember a serving of rice is one-third of a cup! Ask for a to-go box before your meal, and store away the extra portions for another meal. It's usually a good idea to order fewer dishes than people and then share them family style.

Choose the following dishes more often:
- ✓ Dishes with steamed rice or noodles.
- ✓ Steamed fish, stir-fried chicken or other lean meats.
- ✓ Stir-fried dishes with fresh vegetables such as broccoli, cabbage, carrots, water chestnuts, mushrooms and sprouts. Try tofu!
- ✓ For dessert, have the fortune cookie if you want. Coconut desserts can be high in fat and calories.

Choose the following dishes less often:

- ✓ Fried rice, noodles, egg rolls and wonton.
- ✓ Breaded and fried meats found in tempura or sweet-and-sour sauce. Ask how the meat is prepared before ordering.
- ✓ Dishes with cashews or peanuts—ask that the amount of nuts be cut in half.

MORE HELPFUL TIPS

🍎 **Let family or friends who are dining with you know that you plan to eat healthy.** Don't let what others order change your plans for choosing nutritious low-fat and low-calorie foods.

🍎 **Become familiar with a few restaurants you enjoy where you know you can order healthy foods.** Learn to make special requests, such as substituting steamed rice for fried rice. Ask that your meal be prepared with less oil or fewer added fats. Avoid restaurants or foods that can tempt you from your plan.

🍎 **If you order an item that is higher in fat, balance it with a low-fat choice, such as steamed rice or steamed vegetables.**

🍎 **Ask that stir-fry and other dishes be cooked with very little oil.**

🍎 **Be careful when eating Asian food buffet style.** Plan to make healthy choices and select reasonable portions.

🍎 **When eating take-out food at home, serve what you need on a plate and store the rest.**

DINING OUT *DELIZIOSO!*

Italian food is an American favorite! Almost everyone has a favorite little Italian restaurant. Typically serving good food and having quaint atmospheres, Italian restaurants are a great place to fellowship with family and friends. Italian food offers many healthy choices. Fresh breads, pastas and tomato-based sauces are great choices on any eating plan. But depending on how they're prepared, these same foods can be less-healthy choices: garlic bread with butter and cheese, pastas cooked in oil or covered with cheese, cream-based sauces and large portions. Add the cheesecake, and you can easily exceed a day's worth of calories.

A Taste of Italy

You may not speak Italian, but you can learn how to read the menu. Learn these common terms to help you make more-healthful choices:

Low in Fat	High in Fat
Baked, broiled or roasted	*Alfredo*—butter or cheese sauces
Marinara—tomato-based sauces	Cheese- or meat-filled pastas
Marsala or *cacciatore*	*Crema*—cream-based sauces
Minestrone	*Fritto*—fried
Primavera	Garlic bread
Red or white clam sauce	*Parmigiana*

Note: Just because it's green doesn't mean it's low fat! *Pesto*, made with basil, olive oil, pine nuts and grated cheese, is generally high in fat and calories. Use it carefully!

Healthy Choices for Any Occasion

Appetizers

How does hot garlic bread sound? Be careful—a couple of slices can add up to 500 calories! Ask that your waiter not bring the garlic bread to the table, or plan to split a piece with a companion. Dipping your bread in olive oil also adds calories. Ask for bread without the butter, or have breadsticks instead.

Start your meal with minestrone soup or gazpacho and a salad with dressing on the side. You can even make these your main meal. A Caesar salad with eggs, creamy dressing, grated cheese and croutons is generally high in fat and calories.

Do you enjoy antipasto? Antipasto with seafood and marinated vegetables is usually your best choice. Watch out for antipasto with lots of cheese, fried vegetables, meats and olives, all of which can be high in calories and fat.

The Main Meal

Italian portions are often two to three times more than you need. Remember a serving of pasta is a half cup! Ask for a to-go box before your meal and keep the extra portions for another day, or consider splitting a dish with a companion.

Choose the following dishes more often:
- ✓ Grilled chicken breast or veal with marsala or cacciatore.
- ✓ Pasta with marinara or pasta primavera (pasta with vegetables).
- ✓ Clam sauce.

Choose the following dishes less often:
- ✓ Lasagna or cheese-filled pasta (ravioli, cannelloni and manicotti).
- ✓ Italian sausage, pancetta (bacon) or prosciutto (ham).
- ✓ Eggplant or veal parmigiana—breaded and fried.

Pizza

Pizza can be a healthy choice. Here are some tips for ordering:
- **Choose a thin crust instead of thick-crust or deep-dish pizza.**
- **Ask that your pizza be prepared with less cheese (or even no cheese).**
- **Select vegetables as toppings instead of high-fat and high-sodium meats.**
- **Limit yourself to one or two pieces.** For added variety, eat a salad instead of an extra piece.

MORE HELPFUL TIPS

- **Make a plan and stick with it.** Remember your goal of reaching or maintaining a healthy weight.
- **Let family or friends who are dining with you know that you plan to eat healthy.** Don't let what others order change your plans for choosing nutritious low-fat and low-calorie foods.
- **Become familiar with a few restaurants you enjoy where you know you can order healthy foods.** Learn to make special requests, such as substituting tomato-based sauces for cream- or cheese-based sauces. Ask that your meal be prepared with less oil or butter. Avoid restaurants and foods that can tempt you from your plan.
- **When eating take-out food at home, serve what you need on a plate and store the rest.**

DINING OUT—SOUTH OF THE BORDER

Mexican food is known for its hot and spicy flavors. Dining south of the border is also popular for its festive atmosphere. Mexican restaurants offer good times and good food. You might think that Mexican food is off-limits. Actually, the staples of Mexican cuisine offer nutritious choices: chicken and other lean meats, tortillas, beans, rice and salsa. Of course, many also offer less-healthy choices such as fried tortillas, refried beans, too much cheese, high-fat dips and sauces and portions that are too large. Be careful or your food fiesta can easily exceed a whole day's worth of calories and fat!

MENU LINGO

To make healthy choices, you must first learn to read the menu.

Low in Fat	High in Fat
Baked, broiled, simmered or *asada* (grilled)	*Chili con queso* (cheese sauce)
Fajitas (grilled meat and soft tortillas)	*Chorizo* (sausage)
Picante sauce or salsa	Fried or crispy
Salsa verde (green sauce)	Guacamole and sour cream
Veracruz or *ranchero* (tomato-based) sauces	Refried, often with lard

HEALTHY CHOICES

Appetizers

How do hot chips with fresh salsa or chili con queso sound? It's easy to consume 500 calories or more before your meal arrives. Plan ahead to limit the number of chips you will eat (5 to 8 chips are around 100 calories). Better yet, ask that chips not be brought to your table. Ask for steamed corn tortillas instead.

Tortilla or bean soup and a salad are a healthy start to your meal—they can even be the whole meal! Ask for the salad dressing, guacamole and sour cream to be served on the side. Salsa makes a nutritious no-fat dressing. Watch out for taco salad though—particularly if it's served in a tortilla shell.

The Main Meal

Mexican dinners tend to be large. Avoid combination or deluxe plates, and order a la carte or side orders instead. Another option is to split a combination plate with a companion.

Choose the following dishes more often:

- ✓ Grilled chicken breast with rice and vegetables.
- ✓ Fajitas with grilled chicken or lean meat, but watch out for cheese, guacamole and sour cream; ask for extra lettuce, tomatoes and salsa instead.
- ✓ Chicken enchiladas with red or green (*verde*) sauce; hold the sour cream.
- ✓ Bean or chicken burritos made with a soft (not fried) tortilla. Request the amount of cheese to be cut in half.

Choose the following dishes less often:

- ✓ Tacos, chalupas and flautas.
- ✓ Cheese enchiladas or enchiladas with cheese or cream sauce.
- ✓ *Carnitas* (fried beef or pork) or chorizo.
- ✓ Fried burrito or *chimichanga*.

More Helpful Tips

- **Make a plan and stick with it.** Remember your goal of reaching or maintaining a healthy weight.
- **Let family or friends who are dining with you know that you plan to eat healthy.** Don't let what others order change your plans for choosing nutritious low-fat and low-calorie foods.
- **Become familiar with a few restaurants you enjoy where you know you can order healthy foods.**
- **Order a side of Mexican rice and pinto or black beans—instead of refried beans—with your main item.**
- **Avoid restaurants or foods that can tempt you from your plan.**
- **Order a la carte items.** This allows you to pick and choose the foods that are healthiest and that you enjoy.
- **Watch portion sizes.** Ask for a to-go box before your meal or split your meal with a companion.
- **When eating take-out food at home, serve what you need on a plate and store the rest.**

No matter whether it's traditional Mexican cuisine, Tex-Mex or Mexican-American, you can enjoy a healthful meal when eating south of the border. Simply follow four simple guidelines: Have a plan; know how to find healthful choices; order wisely; and eat what you know is best for you.

An Ounce of Prevention

THE TRUTH ABOUT FATS

"Low fat," "fat free," "nonfat," "no fat," "less fat," "reduced fat"—too much fat! Surveys reveal that dietary fat is the number one nutritional concern of Americans. In fact, reducing dietary fat has become an obsession for many. Despite our knowledge about fat and the availability of more low-fat foods, the number of Americans who are overweight or obese is on the rise.

FATS ARE ESSENTIAL FOR GOOD HEALTH!

Fats are an important source of energy. They supply, carry and store the fat-soluble vitamins—A, D, E and K. Fats are involved in the production of nerve cells, cell membranes and many important hormones. Fat helps your body maintain healthy skin and hair. Body fat cushions and insulates the body. Fat also gives certain foods their taste, texture and aroma. Fat satisfies hunger and makes many foods more pleasurable to eat. However, too much fat in the diet is associated with heart disease, certain cancers, diabetes, obesity and high blood pressure.

HOW MUCH FAT DO I NEED?

With fat intake averaging about 34 percent of calories, the typical American diet is still too high in fat. The goal is to keep total fat intake to 30 percent of calories or less. Fat contains nine calories per gram, which is over twice the calories supplied by carbohydrates and proteins. Because high-fat foods contain more calories, they probably increase the likelihood of weight gain. However, too many calories and not enough physical activity are the real problems. Even eating low-fat foods high in calories will result in weight gain.

Variety, balance and moderation are the keys to a healthy eating plan. Cutting fat without cutting calories or without getting more physical activity will not help you lose weight. The Live-It plan provides a healthy balance of fat that makes up between 20 to 30 percent of total calories.

DIFFERENT TYPES OF FAT

All fats are made up of carbon, hydrogen and oxygen molecules and are classified by their chemical structure—saturated, polyunsaturated and monounsaturated. Most foods contain all three types of fats but in different amounts.

Saturated

- "Saturated" refers to a fat that has all the hydrogen molecules it can hold. This saturation with hydrogen creates a rigid structure that is solid at room temperature.
- Saturated fats raise blood cholesterol levels more than any other type of fat. Animal foods such as meat, poultry, fish, butter, milk and cheese are high in saturated fats. Coconut oil, palm oil and palm kernel oil are also high in saturated fat.

Polyunsaturated and Monounsaturated

- Polyunsaturated and monounsaturated fats are not saturated with hydrogen molecules. Because they are unsaturated, they have flexible structures that are fluid at room temperature. Vegetable oils are higher in unsaturated fats.
- Polyunsaturated fats may help decrease blood cholesterol levels when substituted for saturated fats. Common sources of polyunsaturated fats are safflower oil, sunflower oil, corn oil, soybean oil and many nuts and seeds.
- Monounsaturated fats also help decrease blood cholesterol levels when substituted for saturated fats. Common sources of monounsaturated fats are olive oil, canola oil, peanut oil and avocados.

CUTTING DOWN FAT

When it comes to calories, all fats are created equal. Because all fats are high in calories, cutting back on fat can help you consume fewer calories and lose weight—physical activity helps, too! The highest sources of dietary fat are found in meats, cheese, eggs, dairy products, desserts, snack foods and nuts. The key to low-fat eating is learning to choose the foods highest in nutrition and lowest in calories—whole grains, fruits, vegetables, lean meats, poultry, fish and low-fat dairy products. Much of the fat in our diet is added—butter, margarine, cheese, oils and salad dressings. Use less of these fats in cooking and preparation. Also, make the switch to low-fat or nonfat alternatives when available. But remember, not all low-fat versions of cakes, cookies or snack foods are low calorie!

Here are some more helpful tips for cutting down on the fat and saturated fat in your eating plan:

Eat Less Saturated Fat

Saturated fat is the main culprit when it comes to high blood cholesterol levels. Specifically, eating lots of saturated fat will increase the LDL cholesterol, which is the bad cholesterol that's linked to fatty buildup in the arteries. Certain cancers may also be related to higher intakes of saturated fat. That's why it's especially important to limit intake of this type of fat.

Meat is where Americans get most of the saturated fat and cholesterol in their diet—although cheese is a close second. Instead of fatty meats, look for lean cuts of beef and pork, usually labeled "loin" or "round." And look for lean or extra-lean ground beef, chicken or turkey. Buy cuts labeled "select" rather than "prime" or "choice." Remove extra fat and use low-fat cooking methods—grill, boil, broil, bake and roast instead of frying. Look for reduced-fat or fat-free versions of luncheon meats and hot dogs.

More Helpful Tips

- Use all fats and oils sparingly, selecting polyunsaturated and monounsaturated fats instead of saturated fats such as butter, lard, shortening and tropical oils (coconut, palm and palm kernel).
- Drink nonfat or low-fat milk (1%) and choose low-fat or nonfat versions of yogurt and sour cream.
- Learn to modify your recipes with low-fat substitutions.
- Limit the amount of cheese in your eating plan. Choose cheeses with 3 to 5 grams of fat per ounce. Use ⅓ to ½ less cheese than a recipe calls for. You can even mix low-fat and nonfat versions to cut down on fat and calories. Ounce for ounce, cheese is as high in fat and saturated fat as meat!
- Choose low-fat salad dressings and mayonnaise with no more than 1 gram of saturated fat per tablespoon. Choose mustard, ketchup and other low-fat spreads and condiments more often.
- Limit the number of eggs you eat each week to two or three. Or substitute two egg whites for every whole egg—the yolks contain most of the fat and cholesterol—or use cholesterol-free egg substitutes.
- Use low-fat cooking methods: Make low-fat substitutions in your recipes; sauté using low-sodium broth instead of oils and other fats; chill soups and stews and skim off the fat that collects on the surface.
- Cut down on bakery and snack foods—cakes, cookies, pastries, doughnuts and chips. Even low-fat versions can be high in calories!

Note: Children below the age of two should not follow a fat-restricted diet.

ALL FATS ARE NOT CREATED EQUAL

In terms of calories, all fats are created equal—9 calories per gram. The difference is the effect specific fats have on cholesterol levels and other aspects of health. You're probably aware that diets high in saturated fat and cholesterol are associated with higher levels of blood cholesterol and greater risk for heart disease. Certain cancers may also be related to higher intakes of saturated fat. Certain fats—in moderation—may even have beneficial effects on health. Monounsaturated fatty acids in olive and canola oils may increase HDL (*good*) cholesterol in some people when substituted for saturated fat in the diet.

Because not all fats are created equal when it comes to health, it's important to pay attention to the types of fat you eat. No one is recommending that you increase the amount of fat in your eating plan, but it is important to shift the balance in favor of healthier fats.

Experts recommend the following limitations:

- Total fat to 30 percent or less of calories.
- Saturated fat to less than 10 percent of calories.
- Polyunsaturated fat to 10 percent of calories.
- Monounsaturated fat to between 10 percent and 15 percent of calories.

RATING THE OILS

Fats and oils contain a combination of all three types of fatty acids: saturated, polyunsaturated and monounsaturated. All oils are 100 percent fat and contain 120 calories per tablespoon. The following chart compares fats higher in unsaturated fatty acids with those higher in saturated fatty acids:

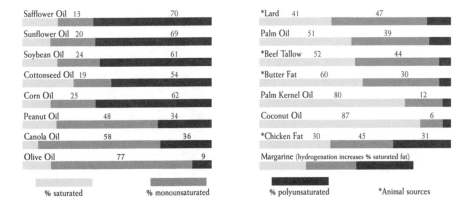

Safflower Oil 13 — 70	*Lard 41 — 47
Sunflower Oil 20 — 69	Palm Oil 51 — 39
Soybean Oil 24 — 61	*Beef Tallow 52 — 44
Cottonseed Oil 19 — 54	*Butter Fat 60 — 30
Corn Oil 25 — 62	Palm Kernel Oil 80 — 12
Peanut Oil 48 — 34	Coconut Oil 87 — 6
Canola Oil 58 — 36	*Chicken Fat 30 — 45 — 31
Olive Oil 77 — 9	Margarine (hydrogenation increases % saturated fat)

% saturated   % monounsaturated   % polyunsaturated   *Animal sources

The following are tips for including fats and oils in a healthy eating plan:

- 🍂 Cut down on all fats and oils.
- 🍂 Choose unsaturated sources of fat more often than saturated sources.
- 🍂 Choose a monounsaturated source such as canola or olive oil and a polyunsaturated source such as safflower or corn oil. Use limited amounts of both in cooking and preparing foods.
- 🍂 Choose soft-tub margarine with liquid vegetable oil or water listed as the first ingredient more often than margarine (with hydrogenated fats as the first ingredient), stick margarine or butter.

FAT SERVINGS

To meet the above guidelines for total fat intake and balance, limit yourself to 3 to 5 servings of fat each day. Choose the following unsaturated fats instead of ones higher in saturated fat. One exchange equals

1 teaspoon vegetable oil	2 to 3 teaspoons seeds or nuts	1 tablespoon reduced-fat margarine
$\frac{1}{8}$ medium avocado	1 tablespoon low-fat salad dressing	1 teaspoon peanut butter
1 teaspoon regular mayonnaise	1 teaspoon regular margarine	1 tablespoon low-fat mayonnaise
5 large or 10 small olives		

Remember: A fat exchange equals 5 grams of fat. Watch out for hidden fats in your eating plan!

HYDROGENATED FATS AND TRANS FATTY ACIDS

You may have heard about hydrogenated fats. Hydrogenation is a process that makes unsaturated oils more solid at room temperature (i.e., more like saturated fats). Hydrogenation also increases the amount of trans fatty acids. Trans fatty acid simply refers to where the hydrogen is placed on the fat molecule. Actually, trans fatty acids are found naturally in many foods such as meat, butter and milk. You will commonly see the terms "partially hydrogenated" or "hydrogenated" vegetable oil on the label of many processed foods such as margarine, salad dressings, crackers, chips and other baked goods. Hydrogenated fats and trans fatty acids can raise blood cholesterol levels but probably not as much as saturated fats. Choose margarine that lists liquid vegetable oil or water as the first ingredient and no more than 2 grams of saturated fat per tablespoon. There is no reason to switch to butter because of health concerns about hydrogenated fats or trans fatty acids.

OMEGA-3 FATTY ACIDS

Omega-3 fatty acids are polyunsaturated fatty acids found mostly in cold-water fish and some vegetable oils. Omega-3 fatty acids may reduce the risk of heart disease through effects on cholesterol, blood-clotting factors and blood pressure. Good sources include salmon, albacore tuna, mackerel, sardines and lake trout. *Eat more fish!* A healthy eating plan can include several servings each week. Canola, soybean and flaxseed oils are also good sources of omega-3 fatty acids.

FAT REPLACERS—FAKE FATS

Fat replacers are added to cheeses, desserts, salad dressings and snack foods to give them the taste and feel of the "full-fat" versions—without the calories! Olestra (OLEAN) is one of the newer fat replacers. Olestra is made from a combination of vegetable fat and carbohydrate. It's calorie free because it passes through the body without being digested. Olestra appears to be safe, but it may interfere with the absorption of the fat-soluble vitamins and cause digestive discomfort in some people. Simplesse is a fat replacer found mostly in frozen dairy products. It's made from protein. Although foods made with fat replacers are low in fat, they still have calories and can be low in nutrients.

As always, moderation, balance and variety are the keys to a healthy eating plan.

CHOOSING HIGH-FIBER FOODS

Many of the foods you eat influence your risk for several diseases, including heart disease, stroke, diabetes and certain cancers. Following an eating plan that is high in fiber and low in saturated fat and cholesterol reduces your risk for these diseases. High-fiber foods may also help you achieve and maintain a healthy weight. Health experts recommend that you eat 25 to 30 grams of fiber each day; the national average is 15 grams or less!

You can get all the fiber you need if you eat a variety of foods, including:

- Six to 11 servings of bread, cereal, rice, pasta and other grains daily. At least three servings from this group should include whole-grain foods.
- Five or more servings of fruits and vegetables daily.
- Legumes—beans, peas, soybeans and lentils—at least once or twice each week.

FIBER FACTS

Fiber is found only in the cell walls of plants—fruits, vegetables and grains. Your body does not digest or absorb fiber. Grains are made up of three parts—bran, endosperm and germ. Most processed grain foods are made from the endosperm. The endosperm contains the energy—carbohydrates and protein—but little of the fiber, vitamins, minerals and phyto-chemicals (plant chemicals believed to promote health). Whole grains also contain the bran and the germ, which are higher in fiber and nutrients. There are two main types of fiber in the diet—soluble and insoluble.

Soluble fiber dissolves in water and forms a gel in the digestive system. The texture of foods like cooked oatmeal comes from soluble fiber. Soluble fiber lowers blood cholesterol levels by blocking the absorption of cholesterol and fats from the diet. It may also have other cholesterol-lowering effects. In fact, scientists have isolated a component of soluble fiber called beta-glucan that appears to be responsible for many of these benefits. Soluble fiber may also help lower blood sugar. Good sources of soluble fiber include oatmeal, oat bran, barley, dried beans, peas, brown rice and apples.

Insoluble fiber does not dissolve in water. Insoluble fiber is more important in digestive health. It provides the roughage that improves bowel function and lowers your risk of colon cancer. Except for being a substitute for foods higher in fat and cholesterol, insoluble fiber does not appear to lower cholesterol levels. Good sources of insoluble fiber are whole-grain breads and cereals, wheat bran and most fruits and vegetables.

DIETARY FIBER AND WEIGHT CONTROL

Both types of fiber may help in weight control. High-fiber foods are more filling and less fattening (i.e., they are usually lower in calories and fat). Also, eating meals that are high in fiber—fruits, vegetables, whole grains and legumes—leaves less room for foods that are high in calories and fat. Very high fiber, low-calorie diets are not good ways to lose weight because they come up short in other important nutrients. Fiber supplements are also not recommended for weight loss. Balance, moderation and variety are the keys to good nutrition!

GETTING ENOUGH OF THE RIGHT KIND OF FIBER

Do you eat three servings of whole grains each day? Experts recommend that at least 3 of the 6 to 11 servings of breads, cereals, rice and pasta that you eat every day be whole grains. White and wheat breads, white rice, refined pasta and many cereals do not count as whole grain. Look for "whole grain," "multigrain" or "whole wheat" on the label. Don't let the names "wheat bread" and "wheat cereal" fool you—these foods are often colored with caramel or molasses. Look at the label—does it contain 2 or more grams of fiber per serving?

What foods can you add to your eating plan to boost your intake of fiber? Sticking with the Live-It plan will give you at least five servings of fruits and vegetables and six servings of breads, cereals, rice, pasta and other grains each day. This should give you most of the fiber you need each day. For extra insurance, make sure that you're choosing several foods that are high in fiber. Review the following table.

Do you eat at least 5 grams of soluble fiber every day? What foods do you regularly eat that are high in soluble fiber?

Food	Serving	Fiber (in grams)	Soluble	Insoluble
White bread	1 slice	Less than 1		
White rice	½ cup	Less than 1		
Refined pasta	½ cup	Less than 1		
Graham crackers	2 squares	2		✓
Broccoli	½ cup	2		✓
Orange	1 medium	2		✓
Whole-wheat bread	1 slice	2 to 3		✓
Whole-grain bread	1 slice	2 to 3		✓
Whole-wheat pasta	½ cup	2 to 3		✓
Bran muffin	1 medium	2 to 3	✓	✓
Oat, oatmeal	¾ cup	3	✓	✓
Apple with skin	1 medium	3	✓	✓
Brown rice	½ cup	3 to 4	✓	✓
Potato with skin	1 medium	3 to 4	✓	✓
Legumes and peas	½ cup	4 to 6	✓	✓
Bran cereal	½ cup	6 to 15	✓	✓

INCREASING THE FIBER IN YOUR DIET

- Choose more whole- or multigrain breads. Look for whole-wheat or whole-grain flour as the first ingredient.
- Start your day with a bowl of whole-grain or bran cereal.

- Try adding ¼ cup of wheat bran to foods such as cereal, pancakes, applesauce, yogurt or meat loaf.
- When baking, substitute whole-wheat flour for half of the white flour called for in the recipe.
- In baked goods, substitute oats for one-third of the flour called for in the recipe.
- Mix at least one-half refined pasta or white rice with whole-grain pasta or brown rice in dishes.
- Increase your intake of beans, lentils, soybeans and peas. Use instead of meat in casseroles or other dishes.
- Add legumes, wheat bran or other grains to soups, pasta, salads and other dishes.
- Leave the skin on fruits and vegetables such as apples, pears, peaches and potatoes.
- Add fresh or dried fruits to cereals and salads.
- Add extra vegetables to salads, soups and other dishes.
- Read food labels. Foods with more than 2.5 grams of fiber per serving are good sources of fiber.

UNDERSTANDING VITAMINS AND MINERALS

When it comes to vitamins and minerals, does it seem that information is changing faster than you can keep up with it? If you're like most people, you probably have many questions: Do I need to take supplements for good health? If so, which ones do I need? How much is too much? Do supplements contain what they say they do? Who and what should I believe?

It's true—recommendations are changing. The National Academy of Sciences is updating its recommendations on vitamins and minerals. You may hear about Dietary Reference Intakes (DRIs), Recommended Dietary Allowances (RDAs) and the Tolerable Upper Intake Level (UL). Now experts are looking at what levels of vitamins and minerals are necessary to both prevent disease and promote good health, and how much is too much. RDAs are the dietary intakes that meet the nutritional requirements of nearly all individuals, and the UL is the maximum safe level of daily intake.

The following tables will help you get a better understanding of vitamins and minerals—what they do, how much is recommended (DRIs or RDAs), common doses in supplements, Tolerable Upper Intake Level (UL) when available and, most importantly, the best food sources (nothing replaces God's good food). When it comes to vitamins and mineral supplements, you have to decide what's right for you.

First Place advises that you discuss the issue of vitamin and mineral supplementation with your personal physician.

VITAMINS

There are 13 vitamins—four fat-soluble (A,D,E and K) and nine water soluble (C and the B vitamins). Compared to the major nutrients—carbohydrates, fats, proteins, and water—vitamins are only needed in small amounts, and they are not a source of energy for the body.

	ROLES AND FACTS	COMMON DOSAGES	GOOD SOURCES
Vitamin A	Maintains healthy cells, skin, and bones; important for vision and immune function. High doses can damage the liver. It's easy to get all the vitamin A you need from a healthy diet.	Women: 800 mcg[1] RE[2] (4,000 IU[3]); Men: 1,000 mcg RE (5,000 IU)—Avoid supplements exceeding the RDA.	Dairy products (cheese, butter, egg yolks); liver; fish oil; fortified foods; and dark green, yellow and orange vegetables.
Beta-carotene (Carotenoids)	Beta-carotene from plant sources is converted to vitamin A. Beta-carotene is an antioxidant that may protect the body from heart disease, cancer and cataracts.	No RDA—Supplements range from 2,500 to 25,000 IU (1.5-15 mg[4]).	Look for fruits and vegetables with orange, red, yellow or dark green color (carrots, sweet potatoes, spinach, red bell pepper, apricots, mangoes and cantaloupe).
Vitamin C	Antioxidant that protects your body's cells. Important for healthy skin, connective tissue, bone, and immune function. Large doses increase the risk of kidney stones.	60 mg—Supplements range from 60 to 500 mg.	All citrus fruits, cantaloupe, strawberries, tomatoes, red and green bell peppers, potatoes and broccoli. It's easy to get what you need.

	ROLES AND FACTS	COMMON DOSAGES	GOOD SOURCES
Vitamin D	Helps your body absorb calcium and phosphorous and build healthy bones. Too much vitamin D can cause kidney damage and weaken bones.	5 to 15 mcg (200-600 IU)—Supplements range from 100 to 800 IU. **UL is 50 mcg (2,000 IU)**.	Vitamin D is formed by the action of sunlight on the skin. Most milk products are fortified. Eggs, fish, margarine and fortified cereals also contain vitamin D.
Vitamin E	An antioxidant that protects your body's cells. It may protect against heart disease and cancer. It's been *claimed* to cure almost anything and slow the aging process.	Women: 8mg (12 IU); Men: 10 mg (15 IU)—Supplements range from RDA to 400 IU.	Vegetable oils, nuts, seeds, salad dressings, margarine, wheat germ and green leafy vegetables.
Vitamin K	Important for blood clotting; a deficiency of vitamin K is very unlikely because your body produces it from bacteria in the intestines and it's abundant in food.	Women: 65 mcg; Men: 80 mcg—No need to supplement.	Green leafy vegetables such as spinach and broccoli, peas, eggs, meat, milk, cereal and fruits.
Thiamin (Vitamin B1)	*All* B vitamins are important for energy production, metabolism and building healthy cells (proteins, blood and nerves).	Women: 1.1 mg; Men: 1.2 mg—Appears to be nontoxic.	Whole grains, fortified cereals, enriched grains, nuts, seeds and meats.

	ROLES AND FACTS	COMMON DOSAGES	GOOD SOURCES
Riboflavin (Vitamin B2)	Same as thiamin.	Women: 1.1 mg; Men: 1.3 mg—Appears to be nontoxic.	Whole grains, fortified cereals, enriched grains, nuts, seeds, meats, dairy products and green leafy vegetables.
Niacin	High doses used *under doctor supervision* to treat high cholesterol levels.	Women: 14 mg; Men: 16 mg—**UL is 35 mg.**	Same as riboflavin, but meats are the best source.
Vitamin B6 (Pyridoxine)	May reduce levels of homocysteine, which is associated with heart attack and stroke. High doses can cause nerve damage.	Women: 1.3-1.5 mg; Men: 1.3-1.7 mg—Supplements range from RDA to 50 mg. **UL is 100 mg.**	Same as riboflavin.
Folate	Very important in pregnancy; may reduce levels of homocysteine which is associated with heart attack and stroke.	400 mcg—**UL for supplementation is 1,000 mcg.**	Same as riboflavin; legumes and fortified cereals are important sources.

	ROLES AND FACTS	COMMON DOSAGES	GOOD SOURCES
Vitamin B12	May reduce levels of homocysteine which is associated with heart attack and stroke.	2.4 mcg—Appears to be non-toxic.	Animal and fortified foods only.
Biotin		30 mcg—Supplements range from 30 to 100 mcg.	Found in a wide variety of foods.
Pantothenic Acid		30 mcg—Appears to be nontoxic.	Found in a wide variety of foods.

Notes

1. mcg = micrograms
2. RE = retinol equivalence
3. IU = international units
4. mg = milligrams

MINERALS

There are probably over 60 minerals in the body. Just like vitamins, minerals play many important roles in the body.

	ROLES AND FACTS	COMMON DOSAGES	GOOD SOURCES
Calcium	Necessary for healthy bones. Plays an important role in muscle and nerve function and blood clotting. Low calcium intake increases the risk for osteoporosis. High calcium intake can cause kidney stones.	800-1200 mg—Aim for 1,200 mg. Supplements range from 250 to 1500 mg. **UL is 2,500 mg.**	Milk and dairy products (yogurt and cheese); dark green leafy vegetables; fortified foods such as juice, some cereals—tofu and soy milk are also good sources.
Chloride	Helps regulate fluid balance; important in digestion and nerve function.	No RDA—No need to supplement.	Salt.
Chromium	Works with insulin to regulate blood sugar. Studies don't support its role in promoting weight loss.	No RDA—Supplements range from 50 to 200 mcg.	Meat, eggs, whole grains and cheese.

	ROLES AND FACTS	COMMON DOSAGES	GOOD SOURCES
Copper	Important in red blood cell formation and is a part of many enzymes.	No RDA—Supplements range from 1 to 3 mg.	Seafood, nuts and seeds.
Flouride	Important for healthy bones and teeth.	Women: 3.1 mg; Men: 3.8 mg—Supplements range from 1.5 to 4 mg. **UL is 10 mg.**	Fluoridated drinking water and seafood.
Iodine	An important part of thyroid hormone which regulates metabolism.	150 mcg—Intakes of up to 2-3 mg appear safe.	Salt, seafood and some vegetables.
Iron	Needed to carry oxygen in the blood; avoid taking supplements with high doses of iron, unless prescribed by doctor.	Women: 10 to 15 mg; Men: 10 mg.	Meats (the redder and darker the meat, the higher the iron), fortified cereals and grains, beans, nuts, seeds and dried fruits.
Magnesium	Important for healthy bones, nerves and muscles; a component of many enzymes.	Women: 320 mg; Men: 420 mg— **UL for supplementation is 350 mg.**	Legumes, nuts, whole grains and leafy green vegetables.
Manganese	Component of many enzymes.	No RDA—supplements range from 2 to 5 mg.	Whole grains, fruits and vegetables and tea.
Molybdenum	Component of many enzymes.	No RDA—supplements range from 75 to 250 mcg.	Milk, legumes and whole grains.

	ROLES AND FACTS	COMMON DOSAGES	GOOD SOURCES
Phospherous	Important for healthy bones and teeth—helps regulate energy and maintain healthy cells.	700 mg: **UL is 3,000 to 4,000 mg.**	Dairy products, meats, legumes, nuts and eggs.
Potassium	Helps regulate fluid balance; important in muscle and nerve function.	No RDA—Supplements may contain 2,000 mg.	Fruits, vegetables and meats.
Selenium	Antioxidant that protects body's cells. May be protective against some cancers.	Women: 55 mcg; Men: 70 mcg.	Seafood, meats and eggs; grains, nuts and seeds may also contain selenium.
Sodium	Helps regulate fluid balance; important in muscle and nerve function. A diet high in sodium may promote high blood pressure.	No RDA—No need to supplement. Limit to 2,400 mg/day.	Salt and processed foods.
Zinc	Important for cell growth, immune function, wound healing and energy metabolism.	Women: 12 mg; Men: 15 mg.	Meat, seafood, whole grains, nuts, seeds, milk and eggs.

SUMMARY AND NOTES

It's important to try to meet your body's need for vitamins and minerals by following a healthy eating plan. If you decide that taking a supplement is right for you, it's best to stick with a multivitamin and mineral supplement that provides no more than the DRIs or RDAs. There is no evidence that taking higher doses of certain vitamins and minerals is necessary for good health. Whatever you do, try not to take supplements with vitamins and minerals in excess of the highest dosages listed in the tables above.

It's important to note that the above common dosages are for healthy adults only; these levels may not be appropriate for children and adolescents.

If you're pregnant, breast-feeding your child or thinking about becoming pregnant, discuss your nutritional needs with your personal physician. The common dosages listed may not be appropriate if you're pregnant or breast-feeding your child.

The above common dosages may not apply to elderly individuals or people with underlying health problems. If you think you may have special nutritional needs, talk with your personal physician before taking any vitamin or mineral supplements.

Many vitamin and mineral supplements list the Percent (%) Daily Value on the Nutrition Facts Panel. Use the tables above when you're unsure about the amount of a particular vitamin or mineral in a supplement.

DIETARY SUPPLEMENTS—MIRACLE OR MYTH?

It seems like every time you turn around there's new information about vitamins, minerals and other supplements. If you're like most people, you may be confused about what to do! What's true and what isn't?

SORTING THROUGH THE HYPE

- There are no miracle foods or supplements. Avoid anything that promises rapid results or a quick fix.
- Ignore dramatic statements that go against what most physicians, registered dietitians or national health organizations are saying.
- Stick to what you know about good nutrition, regular physical activity and a healthy lifestyle. Eating a well-balanced diet that includes a wide variety of foods is the best way to obtain the nutrients you need.
- Your best bet is to avoid anything that sounds too good to be true!

It's true—vitamins, minerals and phytochemicals are necessary for good health and provide many great benefits! However, the true benefit comes from food, not from supplements.

While we all know it's important to eat fruits and vegetables, only 20 percent of adults meet the minimum recommendation of five servings of fruits and vegetables each day. How many servings do you eat? Never substitute other foods for your exchanges of the fruits, vegetables and whole grains that you need to eat. Better yet, get lots of regular physical activity and add a few extra servings. When it comes to fruits and vegetables, studies show that eating seven or more servings a day may offer additional health benefits.

Energy in a Pill?

Not likely! Vitamins and minerals do not supply energy—that's the job of calories from carbohydrates and fats. However, vitamins and minerals are a part of the process of changing the food you eat into energy your body can use. They're also important for many chemical reactions that take place in your body every day. The best scientific evidence suggests that your body uses vitamins and minerals best in the combinations found naturally in food.

Headlines! Headlines! Read All About It!

It seems like new information about vitamins makes the news every month. You may have heard about antioxidants, homocysteine and phytochemicals. The following are brief explanations of what medical science has discovered:

- **Antioxidants**—Three antioxidants are most often in the headlines: beta carotene, vitamin E and vitamin C. Antioxidants help maintain healthy cells by protecting them against oxidation and the damaging effects of free radicals. Free radicals are potentially damaging oxygen molecules that are produced naturally by the body. Some experts believe that environmental factors such as smoking, air pollution and other stressors increase the production of free radicals. Studies suggest that antioxidants in fruits, vegetables and other foods may help reduce the risk of heart disease, certain cancers and a variety of other health problems. Most experts feel that more studies need to be done before specific recommendations for supplementation can be made.

- **Homocysteine**—You may have heard about homocysteine—a protein in the blood. High levels may be associated with an increased risk of heart attack and stroke. Homocysteine levels can be influenced by what you eat. The B vitamins—folic acid, B_6 and B_{12}—help to break down homocysteine in the body. So far, there are no studies showing that taking B vitamins will lower your risk for heart attack and stroke. Everyone should follow an eating plan that has plenty of folic acid and vitamins B_6 and B_{12}. Good sources of these are citrus fruits, tomatoes, dark-green leafy vegetables and fortified cereals and grain products (rice, oats and wheat flour). Eggs, fish, chicken and lean red meats are also good sources.
- **Phytochemicals**—Phytochemicals—plant chemicals—are substances that plants naturally produce to protect themselves against disease. These same compounds appear to have very beneficial effects on our health as well. You may have heard about some of these: isoflavones, sulphoranes, lycopene and other carotenoids to name a few. At this time, there is no evidence that these chemicals can be concentrated in pill form to provide health benefits. Take your phytochemicals in the form of fruits, vegetables and whole grains.

QUESTIONS AND ANSWERS

Do I Need to Take Supplements?

Currently none of the major health organizations such as the American Heart Association, the American Cancer Society or the American Dietetic Association recommend that healthy adults routinely take vitamin or mineral supplements for general health. There's simply not enough information on the dosages or combinations of vitamins, minerals and other nutrients that work best—or work at all!

For the time being, it is best to get the more than 100 vitamins, minerals and phytochemicals your body needs from the foods you eat. Supplements simply cannot recreate what God has done naturally with fruits, vegetables, whole grains and other nutritious foods. Eat a variety of fruits, vegetables and whole grains each day. Balance these foods with lean meats and low-fat dairy products to get the balance and variety you need for a vitamin-packed eating plan.

What If I'm Already Taking Vitamin and Mineral Supplements?

There is no evidence that taking a multivitamin and mineral supplement that does not exceed the Recommended Daily Allowances (RDAs) is associated with any harmful effects. Vitamin and mineral supplements can be an important part of an overall health plan if taking them helps you to live a healthier lifestyle—i.e., eating a healthy diet and being more physically active. However, dietary supplements are not a substitute for eating healthy! Vitamin and mineral doses higher than the RDAs should only be taken after seeking advice from your physician or a registered dietitian. For otherwise healthy people, there is only limited data suggesting advantages for taking certain vitamin or mineral supplements in excess of the RDAs.

Are Dietary Supplements More Appropriate for Some People?

Supplements may be appropriate for some people.

- Osteoporosis, iron deficiency, digestive disorders and other health conditions may be treated or prevented with certain dietary supplements.
- People who follow very low-calorie eating plans or restrictive eating patterns (such as a vegetarian who consumes no meat or dairy foods) may need supplements. However, we do not recommend these restrictive eating plans.
- People who can't eat certain foods may need a supplement to give the body what it needs.
- Women planning to become pregnant or who are pregnant/breast-feeding should talk to their doctor about the need for certain supplements such as folic acid and iron.

PREVENTING CANCER

Scientific evidence suggests that nearly 30 percent of cancer deaths are related to dietary factors. In fact, experts predict that for the majority of Americans who don't smoke, dietary and physical activity habits are the most important modifiable risk factors for cancer. There is little doubt that nutrition plays a role in contributing to and preventing cancer. A definitive answer about the optimal diet for preventing cancer and which nutrients have specific effects is not yet known.

What Is Cancer?

Cancer is a group of diseases caused by the abnormal growth and spread of the body's cells. When these cells grow out of control, they can develop into cancerous (malignant) tumors. Cancers result in death by interfering with several of the body's normal processes.

Many factors contribute to cancer, including heredity, aging, environment and lifestyle. For example, a smoker's risk of developing lung cancer is 10 times higher than that of a nonsmoker. A woman with a mother, sister or daughter with breast cancer has about twice the risk of developing breast cancer compared to a woman who does not have such a family history. Too much exposure to the sun's rays increases the risk for skin cancer. Early detection and eliminating risk factors are very important aspects of preventing cancer and cancer deaths.

Cancer and Nutritional Health

Several groups publish nutrition guidelines to advise the public about dietary practices that reduce risk of cancer. Current recommendations are based on the consensus of hundreds of experts and thousands of scientific studies. The following are consistent with dietary recommendations from the American Cancer Society, National Cancer Institute, World Cancer Research Fund and the American Institute for Cancer Research:

- **Choose most of the foods you eat from plant sources.** Eat five or more servings of fruits and vegetables each day. Especially try to choose dark green and yellow vegetables, vegetables in the cabbage family, soy products and legumes.

  Eat 6 to 11 servings a day of grains including breads, cereals, rice and pasta. Choose mostly whole grains instead of highly processed or refined grains.
- **Limit your intake of high-fat foods, particularly those from animal sources.** Select lean cuts and smaller portions when you eat meat, use low-fat cooking techniques, select nonfat or low-fat dairy products and replace high-fat foods with fruits, vegetables, grains and legumes.
- **Get 30 minutes or more of moderate-intensity activity on most days each week.**
- **Achieve and maintain a healthy weight.**
- **Limit consumption of alcoholic beverages—if you drink at all.**

SCIENTIFIC EVIDENCE

🍎 **Fruits and vegetables contain over 100 beneficial vitamins, minerals, fiber and phytochemicals (plant chemicals), many of which may protect against cancer.** Some of the nutrients that may be specifically beneficial include the antioxidant vitamins, fiber, calcium, folate, selenium, carotenoids, flavinoids and sulfurophanes. Studies show that an increased consumption of fruits and vegetables reduces the risk of certain types of cancer. The evidence is particularly strong for colon cancer.

🍎 **High-fat diets, particularly those high in saturated fats, are associated with an increase in the risk of cancers of the colon and rectum, prostate and endometrium (uterus).**

🍎 **Consumption of meat, particularly red meat, has been associated with certain cancers.** What's the best advice? Limit meat intake to the recommended servings and portion sizes (3 to 6 ounces); choose lean cuts of meat, poultry (without the skin), fish and meat alternatives such as legumes instead of high-fat red meats; and avoid charring meat over a direct flame.

🍎 **Physical activity may help protect against cancer of the colon, breast, prostate and endometrium.** The protective effects may be related to energy balance and hormone levels.

🍎 **Obesity appears to increase the risk of developing certain cancers.**

🍎 **Alcoholic beverages are associated with an increased risk of cancer in the oral cavity, esophagus, larynx and breast.**

CANCER SCREENING

Cancer screening is one of the most important steps you can take to increase your chances of surviving cancer. Regular screening examinations are currently recommended for the breast, cervix, colon, oral cavity, prostate, rectum, testes and skin. Self-examinations of the breast, testes and skin are important steps in detecting cancer early. A regular medical checkup can also detect cancers of the thyroid, lymph nodes, ovaries and other areas of the body. Here is a cancer-related checkup schedule recommended by the American Cancer Society:

🍎 **Breast**—Monthly self-examination beginning at age 20. Clinical examination every three years in women aged 20 to 40 and yearly after age 40. The American Cancer Society recommends yearly mammograms beginning at age 40. Some groups recommend at least one mammogram between the ages of 40 and 50 and yearly beginning at age 50. Talk to your doctor about what is best for you.

- **Cervical**—Yearly Pap test and pelvic examination beginning at age 18 (or with the initiation of sexual activity).
- **Colon and Rectum**—Regular screening should begin at age 50 (earlier in people at higher risk). Tests usually involve a yearly examination for blood in the stool and a rectal examination. Every 5 to 10 years a test to look at the inside of the colon should also be performed: sigmoidoscopy, colonoscopy or barium enema. Talk to your doctor about the screening test and schedule that is best for you. If you have a strong family history of colon cancer or polyps, you may need to begin screening earlier.
- **Prostate**—Yearly digital rectal examination and Prostate-Specific Antigen (PSA) beginning at age 50. African-Americans and men with a strong family history of cancer may want to begin screening earlier. Talk to your doctor about what's best for you.

CONTROLLING CHOLESTEROL

Today, almost everyone knows something about cholesterol. In fact, many people even know their blood cholesterol numbers. However, with what seems like a new report on cholesterol every day, it's often hard to know what to do.

Believe it or not, cholesterol is important for good health. It's used to make certain hormones, it helps digest fat, and it's an essential part of every cell membrane. Your blood cholesterol levels are influenced by several factors: heredity, diet, physical activity, body weight and other lifestyle habits.

The foods you eat can have a big impact on your blood cholesterol level. Eating foods high in saturated fat and cholesterol can raise your cholesterol level. Too much cholesterol in the bloodstream increases the chances that your blood vessels will become blocked with fats, cholesterol and other components. This blockage can lead to heart attack and stroke.

DID YOU KNOW?

- **Cholesterol is not a fat—it's a fatlike substance.**
- **Saturated fat actually raises blood cholesterol levels more than dietary cholesterol does.**
- **Cholesterol is not found in plant foods—fruits, vegetables or grains.** Saturated fat, however, is found in some plant foods: palm oil, palm kernel oil and coconut oil.
- **Your body makes all the cholesterol it needs.** It is not necessary to get cholesterol from food.
- **Children younger than two years of age should not follow a low-fat, low-cholesterol eating plan.** Fat and cholesterol are necessary for normal growth and development and a healthy nervous system.

Understanding Cholesterol Levels

When most people talk about their cholesterol level, they're talking about total cholesterol. The higher your total cholesterol, the higher your risk for heart disease. However, there's more to blood cholesterol than the total cholesterol level alone. Cholesterol is carried in your body in special packages called lipoproteins.

The two most important lipoproteins are *LDL cholesterol* and *HDL cholesterol*. Think of the *L* in LDL as standing for *lousy*. This is the bad cholesterol that tends to block arteries. People who have too much LDL have a higher risk of heart disease. Think of the *H* in HDL as standing for *helpful*. HDL is the good cholesterol that carries cholesterol away from the arteries. People who have a high level of HDL have a lower risk of heart disease.

You may also have heard about *triglycerides*. In your body, fat is carried in the bloodstream in the form of triglycerides. Triglycerides and cholesterol are often carried together in the same packages. High blood triglycerides levels appear to be associated with an increased risk of heart disease in some people.

Know Your Numbers

Do your cholesterol levels meet these recommended levels?

	Yes	No
Total cholesterol less than 200 mg/dL	☐ Yes	☐ No
LDL cholesterol less than 130 mg/dL	☐ Yes	☐ No
HDL cholesterol higher than 35 mg/dL	☐ Yes	☐ No
Triglycerides less than 200 mg/dL	☐ Yes	☐ No

Did you answer no to any of these? If so, you may have abnormal cholesterol levels. If you have abnormal blood cholesterol levels—particularly high LDL cholesterol—experts agree that lowering your blood cholesterol can reduce your risk of having a heart attack. Recent studies show that lowering your cholesterol level can prevent certain types of strokes, too. Talk to your doctor about what's best for you. If you don't know your numbers or you haven't had your cholesterol checked in several years, make an appointment with your doctor for a checkup.

Your Low-Cholesterol Lifestyle

Everyone needs to follow an eating plan that's low in fat, saturated fat and cholesterol and high in whole grains, fruits and vegetables. It is also important to achieve and maintain a healthy body weight—losing weight lowers cholesterol levels. Physical activity is important because it raises the good HDL cholesterol and helps you maintain a healthy weight. Smoking lowers HDL levels.

Choose	Instead of
Lean meats, poultry and fish with visible fat and skin removed.	Fatty cuts of meat, organ meats (liver, kidneys) or other high-fat meats (sausage, bacon).
Three to 6 ounces of meat each day—3 ounces is about the size of an audiocassette.	Typical restaurant-size portions of 8 to 12 ounces.
Fat-free or low-fat milk or yogurt, and some low-fat cheese.	Two % or whole milk or full-fat yogurt, cheese or cheese spreads.
Margarine that lists liquid vegetable oil or water as the first ingredient.	Butter or margarine that lists hydrogenated vegetable oil as the first ingredient.
Vegetable oils (canola, olive, safflower, corn) and low-fat salad dressings or mayonnaise.	Shortening, tropical oils (palm and coconut), mayonnaise or full-fat salad dressings.
Low-fat cooking methods: broil, bake, grill, roast or poach.	Frying or cooking with heavy creams, cheese and sauces.
More fruits, vegetables and whole grains every day.	Meat and highly processed breads, cereals and snack foods.

COUNTING CHOLESTEROL AND SATURATED FAT

Use this table to compare the cholesterol, saturated fat and total fat in various foods.

	Total Fat (g)	Saturated Fat (g)	Cholesterol (mg)
Liver (3 ounces, cooked)	4	2	333
Eggs (1 whole)	5	2	213
*Shrimp (8 medium)	2	1	167
Hamburger (3 ounces, cooked)	17	8	77
Lean beef (3 ounces, cooked)	8	3	72
Baked, skinless chicken breast (3 ounces, cooked)	3	1	72
Whole milk (1 cup)	8	5	33

	Total Fat (g)	Saturated Fat (g)	Cholesterol (mg)
Natural cheddar cheese (1 ounce)	9	6	29
Glazed doughnut (1 medium)	10	2	18
Skim milk (1 cup)	1	trace	4
Whole-wheat bread (1 slice)	1	trace	0
Fruits and vegetables, except avocados and olives	trace	trace	0

* Shellfish, such as shrimp, were once considered off-limits because of their high cholesterol content. However, because they're low in saturated fat, they can be a heart-healthy choice—but not if battered and fried!

PREVENTING DIABETES

Diabetes is a serious disease and is the seventh leading cause of death in the United States. Sixteen million Americans have diabetes, and one-third of those afflicted don't even know they have it! Each year, nearly 800,000 people are diagnosed and over 190,000 deaths result from diabetes. Diabetes kills more women each year than breast cancer. Diabetes is very damaging to the body and is a major cause of blindness, kidney disease, nerve damage and amputations. People with diabetes have two to four times the risk of heart attack and stroke.

TYPES OF DIABETES

Diabetes means that your blood sugar—glucose—is too high. Your blood always has some sugar in it because your body requires a constant supply of sugar for energy. However, too much sugar in the blood is not good for your health. Most of the food you eat is converted into glucose—sugar—for energy. For the glucose to get into the body's cells a hormone called insulin must be present. In a person who has diabetes, either the body does not produce enough insulin or the cells don't use it properly. As a result, blood-sugar levels rise. There are two major types of diabetes.

🍎 **Type 1 Diabetes** is an autoimmune disease in which the body does not produce enough insulin. It usually begins in childhood or young adulthood. Without enough insulin, the body cannot control blood sugar. The only way to survive with type 1 diabetes is to take daily injections of insulin. Type 1 accounts for only 5 to 10 percent of all diabetes sufferers.

Type 2 Diabetes results from an inability to make enough insulin or properly use it—insulin resistance. Type 2 is the most common form of diabetes and accounts for 90 to 95 percent of cases. This form of diabetes usually develops in adults over the age of 45. Nearly 80 percent of people with type 2 diabetes are overweight. Type 2 diabetes is on the rise due to the increasing age, weight and sedentary lifestyles of Americans.

RISK FACTORS FOR TYPE 2 DIABETES

Doctors don't yet understand all the reasons people develop type 2 diabetes. The following factors—many of which can be lowered with healthy lifestyle habits—are associated with a higher risk:

- Family history of type 2 diabetes in a parent or sibling
- Overweight and obesity (ideal body weight ≥ 120% or a body-mass index ≥ 27)
- A history of diabetes during pregnancy or delivery of a baby weighing more than nine pounds
- Low HDL cholesterol (£ 35 mg/dL) or high trigycerides (≥ 250 mg/dL)
- High blood pressure (≥ 140/90)
- African-Americans, Hispanics and Native Americans have a higher risk
- A sedentary lifestyle

DIAGNOSIS

Experts now recommend that adults 45 years and older be tested for diabetes. If you're under 45 years of age and you have one or more risk factors for diabetes, you should also be tested. Early diagnosis and treatment can lower the risk of the serious complications associated with diabetes. The best way to test for diabetes is to have a blood test performed after you haven't eaten anything for at least eight hours. This is called a fasting plasma glucose test. Do you know your blood sugar level?

Risk Classification	Fasting Plasma Glucose Level	My Level
Normal	< 110 mg/dL	
Increased Risk	110 to 125 mg/dL	
Diabetes	≥ 126 mg/dL	

If your blood glucose is normal, take lifestyle steps to keep it that way and have repeat testing every three years. If your level puts you at an increased risk, ask your doctor about further testing. If you have diabetes, you need to take your blood sugar levels very seriously. If you have diabetes, you need to work with your doctor and a registered dietitian to do all you can to keep your blood sugar under control.

PREVENTION

There are several things you can do to lower your risk for type 2 diabetes. If you're at risk, it's important that you do all you can to prevent diabetes. Fortunately, following the First Place lifestyle will help you keep your risk low. In addition to a healthy lifestyle, make sure to get regular medical checkups.

- **Follow a healthy eating plan.** Healthy eating can help to keep your risk low. The most important thing is to maintain a healthy body weight. A healthy eating plan is high in fruits, vegetables and whole grains, and low in foods that are high in fat, saturated fat and cholesterol.
- **Control your weight.** Weight gain is associated with increasing risk for diabetes—the higher your weight, the higher your risk. If you're overweight, a weight loss of as little as 10 percent can significantly reduce your chances of developing diabetes. Achieving and maintaining your healthy weight range will help you keep your risk even lower.
- **Exercise regularly.** A sedentary lifestyle and low level of physical fitness is associated with an increased risk for developing diabetes. Regular physical activity and exercise help your body use insulin and sugar more efficiently. Physical activity also helps you achieve and maintain your healthy weight and lowers your risk for heart disease. Are you fitting in at least 30 minutes of physical activity several days each week?

HEALTHY LIVING

An Ounce of Prevention

Recipe Index

ALFREDO
    Reduced-Fat Alfredo Sauce, 137

ALL-PURPOSE BREADING MIX, 136

APPLE
    Cinnamon-Apple Pork Tenderloin, 85

APRICOT
    BBQ Chicken Breasts with Apricot Glaze, 107

ARGENTINE CORN CHICKEN 92

ASPARAGUS
    Chicken, 100
    Chicken Breasts with Asparagus and Carrots, 109

BAKED
    Cajun Chicken, 94
    Chicken Parmesan, 98
    Quick Baked Fish, 112

Southwestern-Style Baked Fish, 116
Teriyaki Baked Fish, 115
Twice-Baked Potatoes, 127
Zucchini, 138

BALSAMIC VINAIGRETTE, 128

BANANA
    Cantaloupe-Banana Smoothie, 39
    Pineapple-Orange-Banana Smoothie, 39

BBQ
    Beef and Noodles, 75
    Chicken Breasts with Apricot Glaze, 107
    Chicken Salad, 70
    Frank and Beans, 65
    Steak Kabobs, 83

BEAN(S)
    BBQ Frank and Beans, 65
    Black Bean Salsa, 134

Chicken and Green Bean Dinner, 109
Creole Green Beans, 138
Italian Green Beans, 142
Marinated Green Beans, 138
Mixed Bean Salad, 131
and Salsa Salad, 67
Spicy White-Bean-and-Chicken Chili, 91

BEEF
    BBQ Beef and Noodles, 75
    BBQ Frank and Beans, 65
    BBQ Steak Kabobs, 83
    Cheese and Hamburger Casserole, 82
    Flank Steak, 76
    French-Dip Roast Beef Sandwich, 63
    Grecian Skillet Steaks, 80
    Green Pepper Steak, 84
    Grilled Filet Mignon, 79

Ground Beef Stroganoff with
Noodles, 77
Hearty Beef Stew, 83
Hearty Vegetable and Beef
Stew, 81
Kabobs, 79
Mexican-Style Beef and
Pasta, 81
Open-Faced Reuben
Sandwich, 61
Pasta Primavera with Meat
Sauce, 80
Philly Cheese Beef Sandwich, 82
Rosemary-Sage Steak, 84
Salsa Beef and Turkey Loaf, 76
Salsa Meat Loaf, 76
Seared Veal Chops with
Sun-Dried Tomatoes, 85
Steak Tacos, 79
Stir-Fry, 78
Stroganoff, 78
Texas Round Steak, 77
BEET
Pickled Beet and Onion
Salad, 131
BISCUIT
Chicken Biscuit Stew, 102
BISQUE
Egg Salad Muffin with Broccoli
Bisque, 66

BLACK BEAN SALSA, 134
BOWTIE
Chicken and Bowtie Pasta, 104
BRAISED
Braised Cabbage, 139
Citrus-Braised Chicken Breasts
with Capers, 108
Ginger and Garlic-Braised
Halibut Fillets, 119
BREADED, BREADING, BREADS
All-Purpose Breading Mix, 136
Cornbread, 135
Easy Waffles, 36
Italian Breaded Snapper, 118
Low-Fat Pancakes, 36
Raisin French Toast, 35
BREAKFAST
Burrito, 37
Delight, 38
Open-Faced Hawaiian
Breakfast Sandwich, 38
Power Breakfast Smoothie, 39
BROCCOLI
Chicken and Broccoli Frittata,
103
Egg Salad Muffin with
Broccoli Bisque, 66
Salad, 130
Slaw, 132
Tuna and Broccoli Casserole, 120

BROILED
Grilled or Broiled Halibut, 117
Ham and Cheese Sandwich, 64
BRUNCH CASSEROLE, 37
BURRITO
Breakfast Burrito, 37
CABBAGE
Braised Cabbage, 139
Oriental Chicken and Cabbage
Salad, 90
CAESAR SALAD, 129
CACCIATORE
Chicken Cacciatore, 99
Chicken Cacciatore Pie, 106
CAJUN
Baked Cajun Chicken, 94
CALIFORNIA CHICKEN SALAD,
103
CANTALOUPE-BANANA
SMOOTHIE, 39
CAPERS
Citrus-Braised Chicken Breasts
with Capers, 108
CARBONARA
Spaghetti Carbonara, 122
CARROT(S)
Chicken Breasts with Asparagus
and Carrots, 108
Salad, 129

CASSEROLE

Brunch Casserole, 37

Cheese and Hamburger
Casserole, 82

Spicy Eggplant Casserole, 121

Tuna and Broccoli Casserole,
120

CHEESE

Broiled Ham and Cheese
Sandwich, 64

Grilled Turkey and Cheese
Sandwich, 63

and Hamburger Casserole, 82

Lasagna, 120

Macaroni and Cheese, 136

Philly Cheese Beef Sandwich,
82

Quesadilla, 65

Veggie Cheese Quesadilla, 65

Waldorf Salad with Cheese, 67

CHERRY

Pork Chops with Cherry
Sauce, 87

CHICKEN

Argentine Corn Chicken, 92

Asparagus Chicken, 100

Baked Cajun Chicken, 94

Baked Chicken Parmesan, 98

BBQ Chicken Breasts with
Apricot Glaze, 107

BBQ Chicken Salad, 70

Biscuit Stew, 102

and Bowtie Pasta, 104

Breasts with Asparagus and
Carrots, 108

Breasts with Raspberry Sauce,
93

and Broccoli Frittata, 103

Cacciatore, 99

Cacciatore Pie, 106

California Chicken Salad, 103

Citrus-Braised Chicken Breasts
with Capers, 108

Cordon Bleu, 98

Creole Chicken and Rice, 106

Crock-Pot Chicken Stew, 89

Curry, 96

Fajita Dinner, 96

and Fettuccine, 104

Florentine, 99

Fruited Chicken Salad, 68

with Garlic Gravy, 105

and Green Bean Dinner, 109

Grilled Chicken Breasts with
Corn Salsa, 89

Grilled Hawaiian Chicken, 99

Grilled Sesame Chicken, 90

Light Chicken Enchiladas, 92

Linguine, 100

Marmalade Chicken, 88

Mustard Chicken, 93

Oriental Chicken and
Cabbage Salad, 90

Oven-Fried Chicken (or Fish),
94

and Pasta Primavera, 107

Patty Melt, 64

Pita Sandwiches, 97

Quick Chicken Fajita, 66

Ratatouille, 101

Salsa Chicken, 94

Spicy Chicken Stir-Fry
Fettuccine, 101

Spicy Thai Chicken, 95

Spicy White-Bean-and-
Chicken Chili, 91

and Spinach Salad, 70

Stuffed Chicken Breasts, 98

Swiss-Style Chicken, 102

Yogurt Cumin Chicken, 97

CHILI

non Carne, 122

Spicy White-Bean-and-
Chicken Chili, 91

White Turkey Chili, 95

CHIPS

Toasted Pita Chips, 136

CHOPS

Orange Pork Chops, 86

Pork Chops with Cherry Sauce, 87

Seared Veal Chops with Sun-Dried Tomatoes, 85

CIDER
Crock-Pot Cider Pork Stew, 86

CINNAMON-APPLE PORK TENDERLOIN, 85

CITRUS
Braised Chicken Breasts with Capers, 108
Shrimp Salad, 111

COLESLAW (See also SLAWS)
Summer Coleslaw, 132
Southwestern Coleslaw, 132

CONFETTI SALAD, 69

CORN
Argentine Corn Chicken, 92
Grilled Chicken Breasts with Corn Salsa, 89
Salsa, 134

CORNBREAD, 135

CREOLE
Chicken and Rice, 106
Green Beans, 138
Seafood Creole, 115
Zucchini, 140

CROCK-POT
Chicken Stew, 89
Cider Pork Stew, 86

CUCUMBERS
Marinated Cucumbers, 133

CUMIN
Yogurt Cumin Chicken, 97

CURRY
Chicken Curry, 96

DIJON DRESSING, 69

DIP, DRESSINGS
Balsamic Vinaigrette, 128
Dijon Dressing, 69
Orange Poppy Seed Dressing, 70
Russian Dressing, 128
Veggie Dip, 62

EASY WAFFLES, 36

EGG, EGGPLANT
Egg Salad Muffin with Broccoli Bisque, 66
Grilled Eggplant, 141
Spicy Eggplant Casserole, 121

ENCHILADAS
Light Chicken Enchiladas, 92

FAJITAS
Chicken Fajita Dinner, 96
Quick Chicken Fajita, 66

FETTUCCINE
Chicken and Fettuccine, 104
Spicy Chicken Stir-Fry Fettuccine, 101

FILLET(S), FILET MIGNON
Ginger and Garlic-Braised Halibut Fillets, 119
Ginger Salmon Fillets, 119
Grilled Filet Mignon, 79
Indonesian Snapper Fillets, 111

FISH
Ginger and Garlic-Braised Halibut Fillets, 119
Ginger Salmon Fillets, 119
Grilled or Broiled Halibut, 117
Grilled Halibut Steaks, 114
Grilled Swordfish, 118
Grilled Tuna Steaks, 116
Honey-Mustard Pecan Tilapia, 118
Indonesian Snapper Fillets, 111
Italian Breaded Snapper, 118
Lemon Fish, 113
Oven-Fried Chicken (or Fish), 94
Quick Baked Fish, 112
Salmon Cakes, 113
Seafood Creole, 115
Seafood Gumbo, 114
Southwestern Snapper, 110
Southwestern-Style Baked Fish, 116
Teriyaki Baked Fish, 115

FLANK STEAK, 76

FLORENTINE
    Chicken Florentine, 99

FRENCH
    Dip Roast Beef Sandwich, 63
    Raisin French Toast, 35

FRIED, FRIES
    Oven-Fried Chicken (or Fish), 94
    Oven Fries, 127

FRITTATA
    Chicken and Broccoli Frittata, 103

FRUIT, FRUITED
    Chicken Salad, 68
    Salad, 130
    Tropical Fruit Salad, 129
    Tropical Fruit Smoothie, 40

GARLIC
    Chicken with Garlic Gravy, 105
    Ginger and Garlic-Braised Halibut Fillets, 119
    Mashed Potatoes, 126

GINGER
    and Garlic-Braised Halibut Fillets, 119
    Salmon Fillets, 119

GLAZE, GLAZED
    BBQ Chicken Breasts with Apricot Glaze, 107
    Orange-Glazed Sweet Potatoes, 126

GRAVY
    Chicken with Garlic Gravy, 105

GRECIAN SKILLET STEAKS, 80

GREEN, GREEN BEAN(S)
    Chicken and Green Bean Dinner, 109
    Creole Green Beans, 138
    Italian Green Beans, 142
    Marinated Green Beans, 138
    Onion Fan, 119
    Pepper Steak, 84

GRILLED
    or Broiled Halibut, 117
    Chicken Breasts with Corn Salsa, 89
    Eggplant, 141
    Filet Mignon, 79
    Halibut Steaks, 114
    Hawaiian Chicken, 99
    Sesame Chicken, 90
    Swordfish with Oregano, 118
    Tuna Steaks, 116
    Turkey and Cheese Sandwich, 63

GROUND BEEF STROGANOFF WITH NOODLES, 77

GUMBO
    Seafood Gumbo, 114
    Seafood and Turkey Sausage Gumbo, 110

HALIBUT
    Ginger and Garlic-Braised Halibut Fillets, 119
    Grilled or Broiled Halibut, 117
    Grilled Halibut Steaks, 114

HAM
    Broiled Ham and Cheese Sandwich, 64

HAMBURGER
    Cheese and Hamburger Casserole, 82

HAWAIIAN
    Grilled Hawaiian Chicken, 99
    Open-Faced Hawaiian Breakfast Sandwich, 38

HEARTY
    Beef Stew, 83
    Vegetable and Beef Stew, 81

HERBED
    Italian Herbed Tomatoes, 133

HONEY-MUSTARD PECAN TILAPIA, 118

INDONESIAN SNAPPER FILLETS, 111

ITALIAN
  Breaded Snapper, 118
  Green Beans, 142
  Herbed Tomatoes, 133
KABOBS
  BBQ Steak Kabobs, 83
  Beef Kabobs, 83
LASAGNA
  Cheese Lasagna, 120
  Vegetable Lasagna, 123
LEMON FISH, 113
LIGHT CHICKEN ENCHILADAS, 92
LINGUINE
  Chicken Linguine, 100
LOW-FAT PANCAKES, 36
MACARONI
  and Cheese, 136
  Shrimp and Macaroni Salad, 68
MARINARA SAUCE, 135
MARINATED
  Cucumbers, 133
  Green Beans, 138
MARMALADE CHICKEN, 88
MEAT LOAF
  Salsa Beef and Turkey Loaf, 76
  Salsa Meat Loaf, 76

MEAT SAUCE
  Pasta Primavera with Meat Sauce, 80
MEXICAN-STYLE BEEF AND PASTA, 81
MIXED BEAN SALAD, 131
MUSTARD
  Chicken, 93
  Honey-Mustard Pecan Tilapia, 118
NOODLES
  BBQ Beef and Noodles, 75
  Ground Beef Stroganoff with Noodles, 77
OKRA
  Stewed Okra and Tomatoes, 141
OMELETTE
  Spanish Omelette, 38
ONION
  Green-Onion Fan, 119
  Pickled Beet and Onion Salad, 131
OPEN-FACED
  Hawaiian Breakfast Sandwich, 38
  Reuben Sandwich, 62
ORANGE
  Glazed Sweet Potatoes, 126

Pineapple-Orange-Banana Smoothie, 39
Poppy Seed Dressing, 70
Pork Chops, 86
ORIENTAL
  Chicken and Cabbage Salad, 90
  Sautéed Oriental Vegetables, 140
OVEN
  Fried Chicken (or Fish), 94
  Fries, 127
  Roasted Vegetables, 142
PANCAKES
  Low-Fat Pancakes, 36
PARMESAN
  Baked Chicken Parmesan, 98
  Scallops Parmesan, 113
PASTA
  Cheese Lasagna, 120
  Chicken and Bowtie Pasta, 104
  Chicken and Fettucine, 104
  Chicken Linguine, 100
  Chicken and Pasta Primavera, 107
  Macaroni and Cheese, 136
  Mexican-Style Beef and Pasta, 81
  Primavera with Meat Sauce, 80

Salad, 69
Shrimp and Macaroni Salad, 68
Spaghetti Carbonara, 122
Spicy Chicken Stir-Fry
    Fettucine, 101
Vegetable Lasagna, 123
PEAS
    Sautéed Sugar Snap Peas, 140
PECAN
    Honey-Mustard Pecan Tilapia,
        118
PEPPER(S)
    Green Pepper Steak, 84
    Sautéed Squash with Peppers,
        139
PHILLY CHEESE BEEF
    SANDWICH, 82
PICKLED BEET AND ONION
    SALAD, 131
PILAF
    Rice Pilaf, 137
PINEAPPLE-ORANGE-BANANA
    SMOOTHIE, 39
PITA, PITA BREAD
    Chicken Pita Sandwiches, 97
    Roasted Vegetable
        Sandwiches, 121
    Toasted Pita Chips, 136
    Tuna Pocket Sandwich, 61

Tuna Salad Pita Sandwich, 62
Turkey Pepperoni and
    Veggie Pizza, 66
Veggie Pocket Sandwich, 61
PIZZA
    Turkey Pepperoni and
        Veggie Pizza, 66
POPPY SEED
    Orange Poppy Seed Dressing,
        70
PORK
    Cinnamon-Apple Pork
        Tenderloin, 85
    Chops with Cherry Sauce, 87
    Crock-Pot Cider Pork Stew, 86
    Orange Pork Chops, 86
    Tenderloin and Vegetable
        Stir-Fry, 87
POTATO(ES)
    Garlic Mashed Potatoes, 126
    Orange-Glazed Sweet
        Potatoes, 126
    Oven Fries, 127
    Roasted Potatoes, 127
    Salad, 131
    Stuffed Potato, 64
    Twice-Baked Potatoes, 127
POWER BREAKFAST SMOOTHIE,
    39

PRIMAVERA
    Chicken and Pasta Primavera,
        107
    Pasta Primavera with Meat
        Sauce, 80
QUESADILLA(S)
    Cheese Quesadilla, 65
    Smoked Turkey Quesadillas, 91
    Veggie Cheese Quesadilla, 65
QUICK
    Baked Fish, 112
    Chicken Fajita, 66
RAISIN FRENCH TOAST, 35
RASPBERRY
    Chicken Breasts with Raspberry
        Sauce, 93
RATATOUILLE
    Chicken Ratatouille, 101
REDUCED-FAT ALFREDO SAUCE,
    137
REUBEN
    Open-Faced Reuben Sandwich,
        62
RICE
    Confetti Salad, 69
    Creole Chicken and Rice, 106
    Pilaf, 137

RISOTTO

Shrimp and Vegetable Risotto, 117

ROAST, ROASTED

Chicken Broccoli Frittata, 103

French-Dip Roast Beef Sandwich, 63

Hearty Vegetable and Beef Stew, 81

Oven-Roasted Vegetables, 142

Philly Cheese Beef Sandwich, 82

Potatoes, 127

Vegetable Sandwiches, 121

RUSSIAN DRESSING, 128

ROSEMARY-SAGE STEAK, 84

SALAD

BBQ Chicken Salad, 70

Bean and Salsa Salad, 67

Broccoli Salad, 130

Caesar Salad, 129

California Chicken Salad, 103

Carrot Salad, 129

Chicken and Spinach Salad, 70

Citrus Shrimp Salad, 111

Confetti Salad, 69

Fruit Salad, 130

Fruited Chicken Salad, 68

Mixed Bean Salad, 131

Oriental Chicken and Cabbage Salad, 90

Pasta Salad, 69

Pickled Beet and Onion Salad, 131

Potato Salad, 131

Sesame Spinach Salad, 130

Shrimp and Macaroni Salad, 68

Tropical Fruit Salad, 129

Waldorf Salad with Cheese, 67

SALMON

Cakes, 113

Ginger Salmon Fillets, 119

SALSA

Bean and Salsa Salad, 67

Beef and Turkey Loaf, 76

Black Bean Salsa, 134

Chicken, 94

Corn Salsa, 134

Grilled Chicken Breasts with Corn Salsa, 89

Meat Loaf, 76

SANDWICH(ES)

Broiled Ham and Cheese Sandwich, 64

Chicken Patty Melt, 64

Chicken Pita Sandwiches, 97

French-Dip Roast Beef Sandwich, 63

Grilled Turkey and Cheese Sandwich, 63

Open-Faced Hawaiian Breakfast Sandwich, 62

Open-Faced Reuben Sandwich, 62

Philly Cheese Beef Sandwich, 82

Roasted Vegetable Sandwiches, 121

Tuna Pocket Sandwich, 61

Tuna Salad Pita Sandwich, 62

Veggie Pocket Sandwich, 61

SAUCE

Chicken Breasts with Raspberry Sauce, 93

Marinara Sauce, 135

Pasta Primavera with Meat Sauce, 80

Pork Chops with Cherry Sauce, 87

Reduced-Fat Alfredo Sauce, 137

SAUSAGE

Seafood and Turkey Sausage Gumbo, 110

SAUTÉED

Oriental Vegetables, 140

Spinach, 139

Squash with Peppers, 139

Sugar Snap Peas, 140

SCALLOPS
  Parmesan, 113
  Steamed Shrimp and
    Scallops, 112
SEAFOOD
  Citrus Shrimp Salad, 111
  Creole, 115
  Ginger and Garlic-Braised
    Halibut Fillets, 119
  Ginger Salmon Fillets, 119
  Grilled or Broiled Halibut, 117
  Grilled Halibut Steaks, 114
  Grilled Swordfish with
    Oregano, 118
  Grilled Tuna Steaks, 116
  Gumbo, 114
  Honey-Mustard Pecan Tilapia,
    118
  Indonesian Snapper Fillets, 111
  Italian Breaded Snapper, 118
  Lemon Fish, 113
  Oven-Fried Chicken (or Fish),
    94
  Quick Baked Fish, 112
  Salmon Cakes, 113
  Scallops Parmesan, 113
  Shrimp Cocktail, 116
  Shrimp and Macaroni Salad, 68
  Shrimp Scampi, 109

Shrimp and Vegetable Risotto,
  117
Southwestern Snapper, 110
Southwestern-Style Baked Fish,
  116
Steamed Shrimp and Scallops,
  112
Teriyaki Baked Fish, 115
Tuna and Broccoli Casserole,
  120
and Turkey Sausage Gumbo,
  110
SEARED VEAL CHOPS WITH
SUN DRIED TOMATOES, 85
SESAME
  Grilled Sesame Chicken, 90
  Spinach Salad, 130
SHRIMP
  Citrus Shrimp Salad, 111
  Cocktail, 116
  and Macaroni Salad, 68
  Scampi, 109
  Seafood and Turkey Sausage
    Gumbo, 110
  Steamed Shrimp and Scallops,
    112
  and Vegetable Risotto, 117
SIRLOIN
  Beef Stir-Fry, 78
  Beef Kabobs, 79

Beef Stroganoff, 78
SLAWS
  Broccoli Slaw, 132
  Southwestern Coleslaw, 132
  Summer Coleslaw, 132
SMOKED TURKEY
QUESADILLAS, 91
SMOOTHIES
  Cantaloupe-Banana Smoothie,
    39
  Pineapple-Orange-Banana
    Smoothie, 39
  Power Breakfast Smoothie, 39
  Tropical Fruit Smoothie, 40
  Yogurt Smoothie, 40
SNAPPER
  Indonesian Snapper Fillets, 111
  Italian Breaded Snapper, 118
  Southwestern Snapper, 110
SOUTHWESTERN
  Coleslaw, 132
  Snapper, 110
  Style Baked Fish, 116
SPAGHETTI CARBONARA, 122
SPANISH OMELETTE, 38
SPICY
  Chicken Stir-Fry Fettuccine,
    101
  Eggplant Casserole, 121

Thai Chicken, 95
White-Bean-and-Chicken
    Chili, 91
SPINACH
    Chicken and Spinach Salad, 70
    Sautéed Spinach, 139
    Sesame Spinach Salad, 130
SQUASH
    Baked Zucchini, 138
    Creole Zucchini, 140
    Sautéed Squash with Peppers,
        139
STEAK(S)
    BBQ Steak Kabobs, 83
    Flank Steak, 76
    Grecian Skillet Steaks, 80
    Green Pepper Steak, 84
    Grilled Filet Mignon, 79
    Grilled Halibut Steaks, 114
    Grilled Tuna Steaks, 116
    Rosemary-Sage Steak, 84
    Tacos, 79
    Texas Round Steak, 77
    Turkey Steaks, 88
STEAMED SHRIMP AND
    SCALLOPS, 112
STEW, STEWED
    Chicken Biscuit Stew, 102
    Crock-Pot Chicken Stew, 89

Crock-Pot Cider Pork Stew, 86
Hearty Beef Stew, 83
Hearty Vegetable and Beef
    Stew, 81
Okra and Tomatoes, 141
STIR-FRY
    Beef Stir-Fry, 78
    Pork Tenderloin and Vegetable
        Stir-Fry, 87
    Spicy Chicken Stir-Fry
        Fettuccine, 101
STROGANOFF
    Beef Stroganoff, 78
    Ground Beef Stroganoff
        with Noodles, 77
STUFFED
    Stuffed Chicken Breasts, 98
    Stuffed Potato, 64
SUMMER COLESLAW, 132
SWISS-STYLE CHICKEN, 102
SWORDFISH
    Grilled Swordfish with
        Oregano, 118
TACOS
    Steak Tacos, 79
TENDERLOIN
    Cinnamon-Apple Pork
        Tenderloin, 85

Pork Tenderloin and Vegetable
    Stir-Fry, 87
TERIYAKI BAKED FISH, 115
TEXAS ROUND STEAK, 77
THAI
    Spicy Thai Chicken, 95
TILAPIA
    Honey-Mustard Pecan Tilapia,
        118
TOAST, TOASTED
    Pita Chips, 136
    Raisin French Toast, 35
TOMATOES
    Italian Herbed Tomatoes, 133
    Seared Veal Chops with
        Sun-Dried Tomatoes, 85
    Stewed Okra and Tomatoes,
        141
TROPICAL
    Fruit Salad, 129
    Fruit Smoothie, 40
TUNA
    and Broccoli Casserole, 120
    Grilled Tuna Steaks, 116
    Pocket Sandwich, 61
    Salad Pita Sandwich, 62
TURKEY
    Pepperoni and Veggie Pizza,
        66

EATING HEALTHY, EATING RIGHT

Recipe Index

Salsa Beef and Turkey Loaf, 76
Seafood and Turkey Sausage
    Gumbo, 110
Smoked Turkey Quesadillas, 91
Steaks, 88
White Turkey Chili, 95
TWICE-BAKED POTATOES, 127
VEAL
    Seared Veal Chops with
        Sun-Dried Tomatoes, 85
VEGETABLE DISHES, VEGGIE
    Baked Zucchini, 138
    Braised Cabbage, 139
    Broccoli Salad, 130
    Broccoli Slaw, 132
    Carrot Salad, 129
    Chili *non* Carne, 122
    Creole Green Beans, 138
    Creole Zucchini, 140
    Garlic Mashed Potatoes, 126
    Green-Onion Fan, 119
    Grilled Eggplant, 141
    Hearty Vegetable and Beef
        Stew, 81
    Italian Green Beans, 142
    Lasagna, 123
    Marinated Cucumbers, 133
    Marinated Green Beans, 138
    Medley, 141
    Mixed Bean Salad, 131

Orange-Glazed Sweet
    Potatoes, 126
Oven-Roasted Vegetables, 142
Pickled Beet and Onion Salad,
    131
Pocket Sandwich, 61
Pork Tenderloin and
    Vegetable Stir-Fry, 87
Potato Salad, 131
Roasted Vegetable Sandwiches,
    121
Sautéed Oriental Vegetables,
    140
Sautéed Spinach, 139
Sautéed Squash with Peppers,
    139
Sautéed Sugar Snap Peas, 140
Sesame Spinach Salad, 130
Shrimp and Vegetable Risotto,
    117
Spicy Eggplant Casserole, 121
Stewed Okra and Tomatoes, 141
Stuffed Potato, 64
Summer Coleslaw, 132
Southwestern Coleslaw, 132
Twice-Baked Potatoes, 127
Veggie Cheese Quesadilla, 65
Veggie Dip, 62
Veggie Pocket Sandwich, 61

VINAIGRETTE
    Balsamic Vinaigrette, 128
WAFFLES
    Easy Waffles, 36
WALDORF SALAD WITH
    CHEESE, 67
WHITE TURKEY CHILI, 95
YOGURT
    Cumin Chicken, 97
    Smoothie, 40
ZUCCHINI
    Baked Zucchini, 138
    Creole Zucchini, 140